O9-ABE-293

THE CANADIAN GUIDE TO
PSORIASIS

KIM ALEXANDER PAPP MD, PhD, FRCPC
JENNY LASS MA, RHN

LIBRARY
MILWAUKEE AREA TECHNICAL COLLEGE
Milwaukee Campus

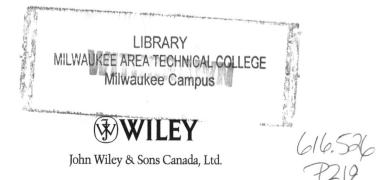

WILEY

John Wiley & Sons Canada, Ltd.

616.526
P218

Copyright © 2011 by SCRIPT Medical Press Inc.

All rights reserved. No part of this work covered by the copyright herein may be reproduced or used in any form or by any means—graphic, electronic or mechanical—without the prior written permission of the publisher. Any request for photocopying, recording, taping or information storage and retrieval systems of any part of this book shall be directed in writing to The Canadian Copyright Licensing Agency (Access Copyright). For an Access Copyright license, visit www.accesscopyright.ca or call toll free 1-800-893-5777.

Care has been taken to trace ownership of copyright material contained in this book. The publisher will gladly receive any information that will enable them to rectify any reference or credit line in subsequent editions.

This publication contains the opinions and ideas of its authors and is designed to provide useful advice in regard to the subject matter covered. The authors and publisher are not engaged in rendering medical, therapeutic or other services in this publication. This publication is not intended to provide a basis for action in particular circumstances without consideration by a competent professional. The authors and publisher expressly disclaim any responsibility for any liability, loss or risk, personal or otherwise, which is incurred as a consequence, directly or indirectly, of the use and application of any of the contents of this book.

Library and Archives Canada Cataloguing in Publications
Papp, Kim Alexander, 1953-
     The Canadian guide to psoriasis / Kim Alexander Papp, Jenny Lass.

Includes index.
ISBN 978-1-118-03828-4

     1. Psoriasis. I. Lass, Jenny II. Title.

RL321.P36 2011   616.5'26   C2011-901084-4

ISBN 978-1-118056-87-5 (ePDF); 978-1-118056-89-9 (eMobi); 978-1-118056-88-2 (ePUB)

General editor and series creator: **Helen Leask**
Editor: **John Ashkenas**
Copy editor: **Gerry Jenkison**
Book illustrations: **Victoria Cansino**
Researcher: **Genie Leung**
Book design and typesetting: **David McFee**
Printer: **Friesens Corp.**
Production editors: **Elizabeth McCurdy, Martha Peacock, Jeannine Rosenberg**

Photographs on pages 13 and 67 courtesy of Kim Alexander Papp; page 16 © D@nderm; pages 17 and 18 © Bernard Cohen MD, Dermatlas, www.dermatlas.org; page 43 © Alison Young MD, Dermatlas, www.dermatlas.org; page 44 © 2011 NZDSI, www.dermnetnz.org; page 76 courtesy of the Phototherapy Education and Research Centre, Women's College Hospital, Toronto, Canada.

John Wiley & Sons Canada, Ltd.
6045 Freemont Blvd.
Mississauga, Ontario
L5R 4J3

Printed in Canada

1 2 3 4 5 PC 15 14 13 12 11

To my spouse, my children and my patients,
each of whom has taught me so much.

KAP

To my parents and everyone who is living
with an illness.

JL

acknowledgments

gnorance begets fear. I must thank SCRIPT Medical Press Inc and Helen Leask specifically for giving the advice, tools, encouragement and information to overcome my fear of diving into this project. John Wiley and Sons Canada Inc. deserves praise and gratitude for their support. Jenny Lass is tireless, persistent, and calm during small storms; I thank her unreservedly. At the inception of my practice two decades ago, I was book smart but knew little about the reality of psoriasis and understood even less. My patients have, day-by-day, educated me about psoriasis as much as I might have informed them. These same patients have helped me understand their disease and suffering. I thank them all. There are a few select and special patients, too many to name but they know who they are, who have given their time, and sometimes their tissues, in a long-time endeavor to find new and better therapies for the life-long disease they share with so many others. The greatest thank you goes to this special group. —KAP

I want to start by thanking my co-author, Dr. Kim Papp, for taking me on as a writing partner. His love of his work, passion for helping his patients and enthusiasm for this project made hard work easier and the long hours worth it. Of course, no book is ever solely the product of its authors, so I want to thank the many people who helped us along the way. Thank you to John Wiley and Sons Canada Inc. and SCRIPT Medical Press Inc for inviting me to be a part of this important project, and thanks in particular to the team that supported me throughout the writing and editing process: John Ashkenas, Helen Leask, Martha Peacock, Abigale Miller and Jeannine Rosenberg. I am also indebted to the experts who donated their time and wisdom to help bring some vital parts of this book to life: J-P Tamblyn of Ahimsa Yoga in Toronto; Dr. Francisco Tausk, Professor of Dermatology and Psychiatry at the University of Rochester Medical Center; Dr. Michael Doyle, Associate Professor and Associate Training Director of the Counselling Centre at the Memorial University of Newfoundland; and Registered Psychologist Beverly McLean in Newfoundland. I'll always be grateful for your generosity—thank you for giving me the tools I needed to reach and help patients better. Finally, I wish to thank my family and friends for their unending support. Thanks especially to my parents, Harold Lass and Diana Papsin Lass, and thanks to Matthew Fitzgerald and Pat Morton, who went above and beyond by helping me with some research when I felt stuck. —JL

Both authors would like to thank the psoriasis patients who so generously shared their stories. Their openness and honesty will allow others with psoriasis to overcome challenges more easily and lead healthier, happier lives.

Finally, publishing specialized but important books such as this is increasingly challenging in Canada. Thanks are due to the following companies who so generously provided grants for the project: Abbott Canada, Amgen Canada Inc./Pfizer Canada Inc. (joint sponsors) and Janssen Inc.

disclaimer

The information in this book may not apply to all patients, all clinical situations or all eventualities, and is not intended to be a substitute for the advice of a qualified physician or other health professional. Always consult a qualified physician about anything that affects your health, especially before starting an exercise program, changing your diet or using a complementary therapy not prescribed by your doctor.

The financial support received from the sponsors of this book does not constitute an endorsement by the authors or publisher of the sponsors or their products. Similarly, the naming of any organization, product or therapy in this book does not imply endorsement by the authors or publisher, and the omission of any such names does not indicate disapproval by the authors or publisher.

contents

Find The Canadian Guide to Psoriasis *supplementary materials online at www.yourpsoriasis.org*

The history of psoriasis ⟶ What psoriasis is, including how it works, where it occurs on the body and what it looks and feels like ⟶ Who gets psoriasis ⟶ What causes psoriasis ⟶ What to expect next

Overview of plaque, pustular, guttate and erythrodermic psoriasis ⟶ Defining mild, moderate and severe psoriasis

The links between depression, cardiovascular disease, metabolic syndrome, digestive disorders, arthritis and psoriasis ⟶ The joints and tissues affected by psoriatic arthritis ⟶ Other types of arthritis

The steps to diagnosing psoriasis ⟶ Medical tests you might experience ⟶ Other conditions that are sometimes confused with psoriasis

Note: All bolded terms can be found in glossary

introduction

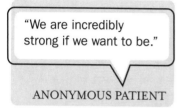

"We are incredibly strong if we want to be."

ANONYMOUS PATIENT

f you have psoriasis or think you might have it, this book is for you. In the following pages we will give you everything you need to know about how to enjoy the best life possible with this long-term, inflammatory skin disease.

We will help you understand what psoriasis is, how it is diagnosed and what kinds of treatments are available. We also offer strategies for overcoming some of the challenges involved in living with psoriasis, such as dating, managing flares and dealing with the many emotions that you might be feeling.

You'll find out about important links between psoriasis and other diseases, as well as how stress and nutrition, might affect you. We talk about the experiences of people who are dealing with this disease at different stages of life and who have health conditions in addition to their psoriasis. You'll also hear from real people with psoriasis and learn how they felt about their lifelong journey with this skin condition. We will even give you tips on how to navigate the healthcare system, how to make the most out of the visits with your doctor, how to find effective and appropriate treatments, and information on what the future may hold for the treatment of psoriasis.

Although we'd love to be able to say that there is a quick fix for psoriasis, the reality is that there isn't. Treating this condition successfully will rely heavily on cooperation between you and your doctor to find what works for you. You need to be proactive in seeking help. In fact, research shows that people with psoriasis are often not satisfied with their treatment. A 2009 Canadian survey revealed that less than half of the people who responded were satisfied with their treatment, and many people with more serious forms of psoriasis were using medications that were probably too weak to help their skin.

We can't cure psoriasis, but we can control it. And the good news for you and the approximately 500,000 other Canadians with psoriasis is that new and better treatments are always being developed. There is also an increasing focus on making sure the needs of patients are met. Therefore, it is our hope that this book will give you the tools and motivation to advocate for yourself so you can find treatments that meet your goals and, ultimately, improve the quality of your life.

Chapter I

psoriasis and you

What Happens in This Chapter
- The history of psoriasis
- What psoriasis is, including how it works, where it occurs on the body and what it looks and feels like
- Who gets psoriasis
- What causes psoriasis
- What to expect next

Psoriasis has been around for as long as we have, but the way it's defined, diagnosed and treated has changed dramatically over time. This condition can occur almost anywhere on the body and usually looks like red, raised patches of skin covered with silvery scales. Sometimes it's itchy and sometimes it's painful. Psoriasis affects 500,000 Canadians and is caused by a combination of environmental factors, genetics and the state of someone's immune system. The course of this disease is unpredictable, but with the right medical help, psoriasis can be managed well.

A Bit of History

Psoriasis occurs only in humans and has probably been around for as long as we have. In fact, some scholars think that this condition makes an appearance in the Jewish and Christian Bible. We know for sure that psoriasis was around during the time of the ancient Greeks, who mistook it for a type of **leprosy.**

By the late 18th century, British dermatologists Drs. Robert Willan and Thomas Bateman had realized that psoriasis was different from other skin diseases, referring to it as "Willan's lepra." The term "psoriasis" finally came onto the scene in 1841 when Viennese dermatologists Drs. Ferdinand Ritter von Hebra and Moritz Kaposi renamed this skin condition, using the Greek word *psora*, meaning "to itch."

Different types of psoriasis were eventually identified over the course of the 20th century, and as we enter the 21st century, researchers around the world are working to find better ways to manage this life-altering disease.

The What and How of Psoriasis

We now know that psoriasis is:
- Chronic (long-term)
- Recurring (it sometimes goes away, but usually comes back)
- Inflammatory (is caused by inflammation)
- Non-contagious (you can't catch it from anyone or give it to someone else)

Psoriasis is generally not life threatening (that is, it very rarely kills anyone), but it can often be life altering and can affect life span. Extensive lifelong psoriasis can actually shorten someone's life by increasing his or her risk of developing **cardiovascular disease (CVD)**, including heart attack and stroke. Psoriasis is also associated with an increased risk of having a few other medical problems, such as depression, **psoriatic arthritis, Crohn's disease and ulcerative colitis** (see Chapter 3). Fortunately, doctors are becoming more aware of the need to develop ambitious treatment plans that aim for greater skin healing and meeting patients' personal **goals**.

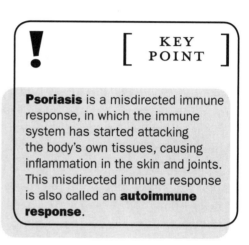

[! KEY POINT]

Psoriasis is a misdirected immune response, in which the immune system has started attacking the body's own tissues, causing inflammation in the skin and joints. This misdirected immune response is also called an **autoimmune response**.

How Psoriasis Works

In order to understand how psoriasis works, you need to know a thing or two about skin. You might be surprised to learn that skin is an organ in its own right—part of a large organ system called the integumentary system, which also includes oil glands, sweat glands, hair and nails.

There are two main layers of skin: the epidermis and the dermis. The dermis is the bottom layer. The glands, hair and nails, as well as blood vessels and nerves, weave throughout the dermis. The epidermis is the outer layer of skin and is divided into five layers of its own. The deepest layer produces millions of new cells every day. These cells are slowly pushed up toward the surface of the skin until they naturally die and flake off. This building or regeneration process gives you a brand new epidermis every 25 to 45 days!

Experts have known for some time that this regeneration cycle goes faster in the **plaques** of a person with psoriasis, creating a buildup of skin cells. With more recent research, these experts now believe that the cell buildup is a reaction to wrong signals from the body's immune system, or defense mechanisms.

Scientists have noticed that the epidermis and dermis of people with psoriasis become flooded with a type of white blood cell called T cells. These cells circulate in blood vessels and are part of the immune system, which allows us to fight off "invaders" such as bacteria and viruses. In a person with psoriasis, these white cells don't do their job properly. Instead, they are misdirected to areas of the skin where they release chemicals that ultimately lead to a plaque forming. T cells jumping into action would be a useful and appropriate response to control a skin infection, but in this case there is no "invader" around to destroy. To make matters worse, special white blood cells that are capable of stopping this kind of misdirected attack appear to be turned off.

It is the combination of the misdirected and the faulty white blood cells that is believed to make psoriasis so persistent and so hard to treat. Therefore, researchers are now focusing much of their efforts on fully understanding why the immune system malfunctions in people with psoriasis and how it can be restored to normal.

What's Happening to Your Skin? [MORE DETAIL]

Healthy skin

Epidermis
(top layer of skin)

Dermis
(lower layer of skin)

Blood vessel

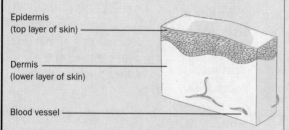

Skin has two layers: the epidermis (the top layer, which is exposed to the air) and the dermis (the lower layer, which contains blood vessels).

Skin in a psoriasis plaque

Flakes of dead skin

Epidermis—thicker than usual

Dermis—more blood vessels than usual

In a psoriasis plaque the top layer of skin is much thicker because the cells multiply faster than in healthy skin. There is also a lot of dead skin at the top, which comes off as flakes. The skin looks red because there are many more blood vessels running through it. These blood vessels come up close to the surface, so it's easy for the plaque to start bleeding if you scratch the flakes away.

What's going on in your plaques?

Immune cells called T cells

Immune **molecules**, such as TNF

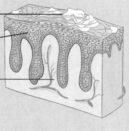

Plaques develop because of immune cells that enter the skin from your blood stream and send the wrong "signals" to the skin cells. These chemical signals, such as a molecule called TNF, cause the skin cells to divide too quickly. They also cause blood vessels to increase in number and branch up towards the surface of the skin.

5

What Does Psoriasis Look Like?

Psoriasis usually looks like red, raised patches of skin covered with white, silvery scales, called "plaques." Psoriasis **lesions** are irregular in shape and their size can vary from person to person. They may be as small as 1 mm (1/16 inch) across, or they may cover your entire body. They also tend be symmetrical (e.g., often, if the left knee is affected, so is the right, and the plaque on the left may be roughly the size and shape of the one on the right).

> "It was weird—if you had a spot on your left leg, you had a spot on your right leg in the same place. It almost mirrors itself."
>
> CHRIS

When a lesion is less than 0.5 cm (1/4 inch) in diameter, it is called a **papule**; a lesion that is larger than 0.5 cm in diameter is called a plaque. The scales on these lesions flake or peel off in small pieces or sheets.

When psoriasis affects the nails, it can take the form of nail pitting, discoloration, thickening, denting, roughness and separation from the nail bed. Psoriasis can also appear as small blisters called "pustules." Don't be confused by this name, though. Psoriasis pustules are sterile, meaning they don't contain live or dead bacteria. This is because psoriasis (unlike, say, acne pimples) is not caused by a bacterial infection in your skin. For a more thorough discussion of the different types of psoriasis, read Chapter 2.

What Does Psoriasis Feel Like?

Psoriasis pustules and plaques can be painful or burn. In some people, psoriasis can also itch. With a doctor's guidance, people with psoriasis usually experiment to find out what works best to make them feel comfortable. However, if the pain and itching are out of control, it's a sign that better treatment is needed.

Where Does Psoriasis Occur on the Body?

Psoriasis can occur anywhere on the body, from head to toe. It can show up on the scalp, under the nails, on the genitals, on the back, on the chest, on the eyelids, on the tongue and gums, and in areas where skin folds (e.g., elbows and knees). Where lesions appear will depend on individual physiology and the type of psoriasis (see Chapter 2).

Psoriasis Statistics: Who Has It and When It Starts

There are 500,000 Canadians with psoriasis. About 40,000 of them are over the age of 70, and 20,000 are children. The first signs of psoriasis usually occur between the ages of 15 and 35 years. Psoriasis affects both men and women. Most people develop **symptoms** before they hit age 30, but there are often hints of psoriasis earlier, even in infancy, that can go unnoticed or misdiagnosed.

Treating psoriasis in the very old and very young can be especially challenging—see Chapters 12 and 13 for information on how to deal with this condition if you or someone you know fits into these age groups.

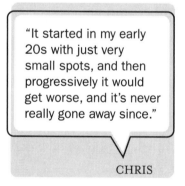

"It started in my early 20s with just very small spots, and then progressively it would get worse, and it's never really gone away since."

CHRIS

The Causes of Psoriasis: A Perfect Storm

There is no known single cause of psoriasis. Experts believe
that three main factors contribute to someone developing this
condition—a so-called perfect storm that can lead to a change in
health: genes, environment and the configuration of a person's
immune system.

There are many different psoriasis risk genes, and they all influence
the odds of developing the condition. A lot of the variation in psoriasis
(how, where and when someone gets it, which other diseases come
along with it, and how someone responds to different treatments) is
probably explained by the complexity of psoriasis genetics.

Some of these genes have been discovered in recent years, and one
is linked specifically to people of Asian and Caucasian descent. Most
people with psoriasis are Caucasian, and 2.5 percent of Caucasian
Americans have the disease. Psoriasis is relatively uncommon in
people of East Asian origin. It is more common in people from
northern China (2 percent) and rarer among people in southern
China (0.5 percent). Psoriasis is very rare in Japan (less than
0.5 percent) and in people in West
Africa and their African-Canadian
descendents.

> "I was born with it. My
> mother had psoriasis
> throughout her young
> life and then when I
> was born, her psoriasis
> disappeared. My
> psoriasis first appeared
> when I was one or two.
> And then it disappeared
> and came back when I
> was about thirteen."
>
> ANONYMOUS PATIENT

This genetic link means that psoriasis
often runs in families. If someone
in your family has psoriasis, you are
more likely to develop it. If one of
your siblings has psoriasis, your risk
of developing it is four to six times
higher than that of the general public.

External triggers, such as injuries
to the skin or infections, also

contribute to the development of psoriasis by altering immune responses. The configuration of the immune system is another factor that influences whether or not someone will develop psoriasis. The immune system is complex and interacts with and affects every organ system in the body, including the skin.

However, it's unclear why some people's immune systems become configured in a way that allows psoriasis to develop. In some cases, we can point to a life event that causes a person's physiology to change and seemingly alter his or her immune system. Sometimes a combination of stressful factors (e.g., chronic stress, poor sleep, poor self-care) acts as a trigger, or a woman might develop psoriasis as a result of the hormonal changes that happen during pregnancy. But most of the time we can only guess why someone's immune system changes at a certain time in life, or why one person's immune response is affected while another person's is not.

Psoriasis is a complicated condition, and we will no doubt discover more about it as research on its causes and effects continues.

Next Steps

If you're not sure whether you have psoriasis, a thorough examination of your skin by your physician is probably all that's needed to diagnose you. Sometimes your physician might also need to conduct a few medical tests, such as a **skin biopsy**, which you can find out more about in Chapter 4.

If you already know that you have psoriasis, it's important to understand that it will likely come and go over the course of your life. It very rarely goes away altogether, except in the case of guttate psoriasis, which often never returns after clearing up (see page 18).

However, more treatment options are now available for psoriasis than ever before, and it is possible to find effective ways to deal with the condition's many physical and emotional challenges.

Taking advantage of the high-quality medical care that exists in Canada is the first step to easing your discomfort, so start by making an appointment with your physician and advocating for yourself by being clear about what you need to live a better life. Accepting the support that is available from patient groups, counselors and your loved ones can also help you deal more easily with the road ahead (see Chapter II and our Resources section for information on finding support).

Although your psoriasis journey may not be easy, know that you're not alone. Many others with this disease have found relief, and so can you.

Chapter 2

the different types of psoriasis

What Happens in This Chapter
- Overview of plaque, pustular, guttate and erythrodermic psoriasis
- Defining mild, moderate and severe psoriasis

There are several different kinds of psoriasis, including guttate, erythrodermic and—the most common—plaque. Each has its own characteristics and challenges. There are also many ways to measure the severity of psoriasis, but what matters most is how much it affects the quality of your life.

Introduction

When people first start to experience symptoms of psoriasis, most feel nervous about what could happen next. They wonder how long their symptoms will last and whether they'll get worse. The reality is, there's no way to tell what course someone's disease will take. However, learning about the different types of psoriasis will help take the mystery out of what's happening and make it easier to talk with a doctor about treatments.

Types of Psoriasis at a Glance

Psoriasis can occur anywhere on the body—it can show up on someone's fingernails or eyelids, or it can cover most of the skin. Common places for psoriasis to appear are the elbows, knees and scalp, and on the back (Figure 2.1). But exactly where the disease shows up and how severe it is depends on the type of psoriasis and how much of the body it covers.

There are several major types of psoriasis:
- **Plaque psoriasis** is the most common. It tends to be a lifelong condition that can affect many areas of the body, including the elbows, knees, genitals, scalp, skin folds, nails and lower back. It rarely affects the face, palms of the hands or soles of the feet.
- **Pustular psoriasis**, another major type of chronic psoriasis, usually affecting the palms of the hands and the soles of the feet.
- **Guttate psoriasis**, which can affect the trunk, arms, legs and face, is usually temporary, but it can be a precursor to plaque psoriasis.
- **Erythrodermic psoriasis**, which appears as severe pustular **flares** that come and go and affect all or almost all of the body.

Figure 2.1 Areas of the body most commonly affected by psoriasis

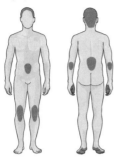

Plaque Psoriasis

About 90 percent of people with psoriasis have plaque psoriasis, which causes plaques that are at least 0.5 cm (1/4 inch) in diameter to appear just about anywhere on the body. The plaques are usually itchy and can range from slightly pink in color to intensely red. They can be flush with the skin or a few millimeters thick, and they can be free of scales or look like clam or oyster shells.

"You get the red patches, then you get into the scaling. I was covered from head to foot. The only place I didn't have it was my face, my hands and the soles of my feet."

MARGIE

Figure 2.2 Plaque psoriasis

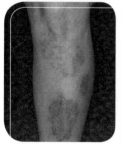

Plaque Psoriasis on Different Parts of the Body

The Scalp

About 85 to 90 percent of people with plaque psoriasis get plaques on their scalp, which is often the first place that the disease shows up. When psoriasis occurs on the scalp, it rarely extends much more than 2 cm beyond the hairline, but it can be intensely itchy and can still cause a great deal of discomfort and embarrassment—more so than on many other parts of the body because it's so visible.

Psoriasis on the scalp usually occurs above the ears or on the back of the head, and it is sometimes confused with another skin condition called **seborrheic dermatitis** (dandruff). It can also often appear around the front of the scalp but is generally less scaly there.

> "It arrived in little tiny patches in my scalp and my forehead, and then it began to travel down my body."
>
> ANONYMOUS PATIENT

The Face

Psoriasis on the face is particularly common in people who have active or very aggressive psoriasis, or it can be a precursor to more severe or extensive disease. Facial psoriasis can take four basic patterns:

- Around the hairline, which can spread to the scalp or face
- Around the eyebrows and eyelids, and in the folds of the nose and lips, with only mild scaling and hardening—this pattern can often look like seborrheic dermatitis and is usually called sebopsoriasis
- Covering the central face
- Over the entire face, which is quite rare and usually happens only in people with particularly aggressive disease

Skin Folds

Psoriasis in skin folds is called flexural, or inverse, psoriasis. Flexural plaque psoriasis is less scaly than other kinds of psoriasis. It's usually found under the breasts, in the groin, in the armpits, in the folds of skin on the abdomen, around the anus, on the genitals and between the buttocks—in fact, many cases of "itchy anus" may be undiagnosed psoriasis.

Flexural plaques are smooth and inflamed or raw, and are less scaly than psoriasis on the trunk or limbs. Sometimes flexural psoriasis around the anus is confused with a yeast infection of the skin, hemorrhoidal itching and pinworm infestations, all of which produce similar symptoms. (To add to the confusion, yeast infections can also affect the groin and armpits, which are common places for psoriasis to appear.) Doctors can determine whether someone has psoriasis or another condition by performing simple tests (see Chapter 4).

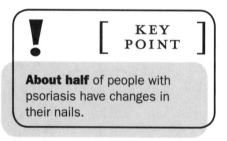

! [**KEY POINT**]

About half of people with psoriasis have changes in their nails.

Nails

Psoriasis under the nails can be quite painful and disabling, in addition to embarrassing. Treatment can be difficult because it's hard to get medicine under the nail bed. Nail psoriasis can show up in a variety of ways, depending on what part of the nail is affected. If psoriasis develops around the nail matrix (where the nail grows from, or its "root"), nails can become crumbly or appear pitted or spotted. If psoriasis develops on the nail bed (the main area of skin under the nail), the nail will probably thicken, and it may separate from the nail bed.

Genitals

Psoriasis can also affect the penis, scrotum or vulva, and looks very similar to psoriasis that appears in skin folds—smooth, inflamed and less scaly. Psoriasis usually stays on the outside of the genitals, leaving the vagina and urethra untouched.

Palms of the Hands and Bottoms of the Feet

Plaque psoriasis on the palms of the hands and bottoms of the feet, called palmoplantar psoriasis, can be very disabling. It's common for this type of psoriasis to develop on the parts of the feet that experience a lot of rubbing or contact with the floor, as physical trauma of all kinds (including pressure and scratching) can cause plaques to form. Unfortunately, plaques on the feet can make standing and walking painful.

Figure 2.3 Palmoplantar psoriasis

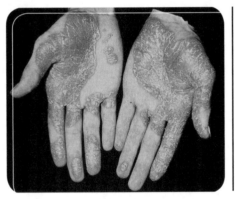

Pustular Psoriasis

Pustular psoriasis looks like small, raised pustules filled with non-infectious fluid surrounded by red skin. It can be triggered by stress, smoking, infections and certain medications. The blisters are painful or itchy, and they can develop in new patches alongside existing psoriasis or alone.

There are two kinds of pustular psoriasis: localized and generalized. Localized is more common, affecting the palms of the hands, the soles of the feet and occasionally other areas of skin. It can make getting around and performing everyday tasks very difficult. Generalized pustular psoriasis, which can cover large areas of the body, is considered a severe flare and may require hospitalization until it's under control.

> "You can't even walk. Your feet blister and your hands get so encrusted. Your hand just keeps peeling. You're shedding everywhere."
>
> ANONYMOUS PATIENT

Figure 2.4 Pustular psoriasis

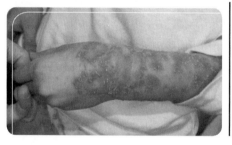

Guttate Psoriasis

Guttate psoriasis appears suddenly, often showing up 2 to 4 weeks after a bout of strep throat or a streptococcal skin infection. It can be confused with or may coexist with a common kind of dermatitis called dyshidrosis, which causes very itchy, small, clear blisters to form on the fingers and palms of the hands or on the toes and soles of the feet. After a few days, the blisters turn white.

You know that you have guttate psoriasis and not dyshidrosis if you develop small papules (lesions that are less than 1 cm or 1/2 inch in diameter) on your trunk, arms, legs and face. This type of psoriasis is usually seen in children and teenagers. People with guttate psoriasis often recover fully after a few days to weeks without treatment, although a short course of **phototherapy** is sometimes recommended. The guttate psoriasis may never return after it has cleared, but at some later time the person may go on to develop plaque psoriasis.

Figure 2.5 Guttate psoriasis

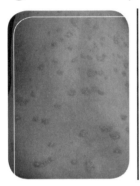

Erythrodermic Psoriasis

Although it occurs rarely, it's possible to experience an episode of erythrodermic psoriasis, a severe kind of flare that usually affects over 80 percent of the skin's surface.

In erythrodermic psoriasis, the skin becomes red, itchy and swollen, although with very little scaling. Sometimes pustules will form and ooze pus, and symptoms can include chills and fever. It may be hard to maintain normal fluid levels and body temperature, and the heart rate may increase because of the large amount of blood flowing through the skin. Normally, 10 to 15 percent of a person's blood flows through the skin, but in erythrodermic psoriasis, it can be as high as 85 to 90 percent.

People with erythrodermic psoriasis might be hospitalized, but they can also be treated at home. They are encouraged to keep warm and supplement their diet with vitamins and minerals, because the rapid growth of skin can deplete the body of essential nutrients.

> "There were times when I had to be in the hospital because from head to toe I was covered. Imagine someone who's sunburned—now imagine that head to toe. You peel and every 2 to 3 hours you lose a layer."
>
> ANONYMOUS PATIENT

Psoriasis Severity: Your Opinion Counts

Although the medical world has created definitions for "**mild**," "**moderate**" and "**severe**" **psoriasis** for the sake of conducting studies, how people with psoriasis define their disease varies quite a bit. At the end of the day, severity depends partly on how much the individual feels the condition affects his or her life and the kinds of treatments that are needed to control it (see A Word from Dr. Papp on page 21).

Scientific studies about psoriasis use rating scales to measure how much of the body is covered by psoriasis, how much relief someone is getting from a new treatment and how much his or her skin condition is affecting quality of life. Your doctor may use some of these measurements as well — he or she has plenty to choose from:

- **Body Surface Area (BSA)**: The BSA is simply a measure of what percentage of the body is affected by psoriasis.
- **Psoriasis Area and Severity Index (PASI)**: The PASI score allows doctors to score the thickness, redness and scaling of psoriasis, as well as how much body surface is affected, and in which areas. Scores range from 0 (no disease) to 72 (worst disease).

- **PASI Change**: The PASI change tracks how much someone's psoriasis has changed in severity. For example, a PASI-75 means that a person's PASI score has declined by 75 percent (e.g., from 12 to 3), while a PASI-125 indicates a PASI score increase of 25 percent (e.g., from 8 to 10).
- **Physician's Global Assessment (static PGA and dynamic PGA)**: The static PGA assesses how severe someone's disease is at one point in time. The dynamic PGA assesses response to treatment. These measures are not of much use scientifically because they can't be precisely defined or measured.
- **Dermatology Life Quality Index (DLQI)**: The DLQI score is based on a questionnaire that allows someone to rank the level of itch, pain and feelings of embarrassment/self-consciousness; note any problems with treatment; and rate how much he or she feels the condition is interfering with daily activities, relationships and sex. Scores range from 0 (no impairment) to 30 (worst impairment).
- **Short Form (SF-36) Health Survey**: This is a general quality-of-life rating tool that is not specific to psoriasis or dermatology. It asks a person to rank how much psoriasis affects his or her life.

A Word from Dr. Papp

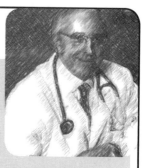

A Word About Mild, Moderate and Severe Psoriasis

Terms like "mild," "moderate" and "severe" are all relative.

Your doctor might consider the small patch of psoriasis on your back mild, but if you're a competitive figure skater who can't find a costume to cover up your plaques, your disease is suddenly a much bigger problem. A very young person with extensive psoriasis will have many social, psychological and physical hurdles to overcome, and anyone whose condition clears up and then returns can feel devastated. So the severity of your psoriasis depends on how much of a problem you feel it is, where it is, how much of your body it covers and the kinds of treatments that are needed to control it.

I usually consider my patients' psoriasis mild if it has only a small impact on their quality of life and can be controlled with simple **topical treatments** such as moisturizers, steroid cream or tar-based products. Most people with psoriasis fall into this category.

You most likely have moderate psoriasis if your disease isn't controlled well with topical treatments. Severe psoriasis usually covers a large part of your body and significantly affects your quality of life and ability to function normally—for example, you might have trouble working or walking. Not everyone is comfortable with the treatments for moderate and severe psoriasis, so it's up to you and your healthcare team to decide which therapies are right for you.

The bottom line is, regardless of what you score on the severity rating scales, what matters most is how your psoriasis affects you and how hard you think it is to control. Surveys and numbers don't paint the whole picture in this complicated disease. If you think that your doctor's assessment of your condition's severity doesn't reflect the reality of your experience, talk to him or her so you can work on finding a more effective treatment plan. There are lots of good therapies out there!

Chapter 3

other conditions that travel with psoriasis

What Happens in This Chapter
- The links between depression, cardiovascular disease, metabolic syndrome, digestive disorders, arthritis and psoriasis
- The joints and tissues affected by psoriatic arthritis
- Other types of arthritis

A few other conditions tend to travel with psoriasis: depression, cardiovascular disease, metabolic syndrome, digestive disorders and psoriatic arthritis. While depression is related to the many psychological challenges that come with psoriasis, the other diseases are either linked genetically to psoriasis or share a similar inflammatory mechanism. Fortunately, there are ways to treat all of these tag-along conditions.

Introduction

One of the curious and frustrating things about psoriasis is that it is associated with other conditions, many of which are linked to chronic inflammation in the body, such as diseases of the heart and arteries, digestive problems or psoriatic arthritis. People with psoriasis are also more likely to be depressed or anxious.

Of course, lots of people can be depressed or suffer from **arthritis**, even if they don't have psoriasis. But when these conditions show up in someone who does have psoriasis, it may not be just a matter of chance—doctors believe that these diseases are linked. For example, a gene called HLA-C seems to increase the risk of developing psoriasis, arthritis and/or Crohn's disease, an **inflammatory bowel disease** discussed later in this chapter.

But keep in mind that you may never develop any of these tag-along conditions, and even if you do, there are ways to treat them, although your doctor may need to refer you to a specialist for appropriate help.

Depression and Psoriasis

Because psoriasis presents many challenges in addition to its physical discomfort, it is understandable that people with this condition might sometimes feel depressed or anxious. In fact, in a 2007 online survey of 514 people with psoriasis, 66 percent reported feeling self-conscious, 56 percent reported feeling embarrassed and 91 percent said that they experienced emotional suffering as a result of their condition. On top of the social stresses a person with psoriasis can face, the disease can become a financial strain, which surely doesn't help when someone is already feeling depressed (see More Detail box on page 25).

People with psoriasis are also sometimes discriminated against or rejected in social situations because of the way their skin looks. A 1993 New York–based study run by researchers at Columbia University revealed that 19 of the 100 adults they talked to who had moderate to severe psoriasis reported having been rejected outright because of their disease, including having been asked to leave a public space such as a gym or swimming pool.

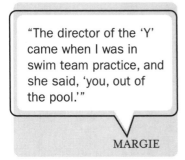

"The director of the 'Y' came when I was in swim team practice, and she said, 'you, out of the pool.'"

MARGIE

While men with psoriasis tend to face greater stress around work, women seem to be more affected by the psychological pressures of having psoriasis—one U.S. telephone survey found that 20 percent of women and 11 percent of men with psoriasis were depressed. A 2007 Canadian phone survey echoed this finding: women were far more likely to say that their psoriasis was a substantial problem in their everyday life.

Socially, teenagers and young adults seem to suffer most. In 1995, a team of psychiatrists at the University of Michigan surveyed over 200 people with psoriasis, ranging in age from 19 to 87 years. The psychiatrists found that the stigma of the condition can affect the ability of younger people to form a positive body image, create strong social networks and build a career.

More Studies on the Challenges of Psoriasis

[**MORE DETAIL**]

- A team of psychiatrists at the University of Western Ontario studied more than 1300 people with moderate to severe psoriasis in 1998 and found that 26 percent of them reported that people purposely avoided touching them.
- Researchers at the same university found in 1997 that 41 percent of the people they surveyed said their sexual activity had declined since they were diagnosed with psoriasis— 60 percent of them felt that their disease was to blame.
- A 1997 study conducted by a team of dermatologists in North Carolina showed that nearly 60 percent of people with psoriasis that they surveyed had trouble finding or keeping a job because of the effects of their disease or its treatment.

However, there may be more to depression in people with psoriasis than the toll it can take on their personal or professional life. Within the last few years, the medical community has started to notice a connection between inflammation and mood. Inflammatory chemicals that are released in someone with psoriasis may travel to the central nervous system and cause impaired physical movement, depression, fatigue, poor sleep quality and inability to think clearly.

One study published in 2006 in the medical journal *The Lancet* found that a powerful anti-inflammatory psoriasis drug called etanercept (see page 89) improved the mood of the people who took it, even when their skin didn't clear up completely. However, it's possible that more subtle symptoms, such as low-level joint pain, could have been eliminated by the etanercept, causing an improvement in mood. This area of research is relatively new, and scientists need a lot more time to explore it before they decide whether etanercept can be used to potentially treat or prevent depression in people with psoriasis.

Continued public education, more studies on the link between inflammation and depression, and providing better emotional support for people with psoriasis are essential to reducing the emotional toll that this disease takes. Improving communication between patients and doctors is also key. Doctors are being encouraged to become more aware of the level of happiness of their patients with psoriasis, and patients are being encouraged to talk more about their emotions.

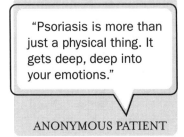

"Psoriasis is more than just a physical thing. It gets deep, deep into your emotions."

ANONYMOUS PATIENT

Cardiovascular Disease and Psoriasis

People with psoriasis run a higher risk of developing conditions that are related to inflammation, such as diseases of the heart and blood vessels. These conditions are collectively called cardiovascular disease. In cardiovascular disease, the arteries that feed the heart become hardened and blocked. This can increase the likelihood of having a heart attack.

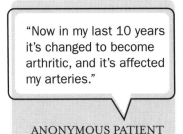

"Now in my last 10 years it's changed to become arthritic, and it's affected my arteries."

ANONYMOUS PATIENT

The worse someone's psoriasis is, the higher the risk of having cardiovascular disease, particularly if he or she is young. For example, some people with psoriasis under the age of 40 have had "silent" heart attacks that are detectable with an electrocardiogram but unknown to them. Researchers are hoping to figure out whether early and effective treatment for psoriasis could help reduce heart attack risk.

It's also possible to develop "**metabolic syndrome**," a term used to describe a group of symptoms that occur at the same time and are genetically associated with psoriasis (see the next section). Metabolic syndrome further increases a person's risk of developing cardiovascular disease. It also puts him or her at risk of having a stroke or developing diabetes.

That's why it's really important for people with psoriasis to take good care of themselves. Read Chapters 8, 10 and 11 to learn how to eat well, deal better with stress and stay fit.

Metabolic Syndrome and Psoriasis

As we mentioned in the previous section, people with psoriasis also have an increased tendency to develop metabolic syndrome. This is a combination of several different conditions that are all bad for the health of the heart: **obesity**, high **cholesterol**, high **blood pressure**, elevated insulin levels and **diabetes**. You're probably familiar with some of these terms, but what do they actually mean?

Obesity
Obesity is when someone has an excessive amount of body fat. Doctors consider a person obese if he or she scores at least 30 on the Body Mass Index, or BMI. This assessment tool takes into account height and weight to come up with a number that indicates whether someone is obese, overweight, underweight or a normal weight.

High Cholesterol
Cholesterol has a bad reputation, but, in the right amounts, it is actually crucial for our health. It is responsible for producing **hormones**, synthesizing vitamin D, forming cell membranes and helping with fat digestion. Cholesterol travels through the blood

stream by hitching a ride on either high-density lipoproteins (HDL), which carry cholesterol toward the liver, or low-density lipoproteins (LDL), which carry cholesterol away from the liver to cells in the body.

People with psoriasis can sometimes develop high cholesterol before they develop skin symptoms. If you have been told that you need to watch your cholesterol, it usually means that your LDL ("bad cholesterol") is raised or your HDL ("good cholesterol") is low, or both. In Canada, the ideal LDL target level for someone who is at risk of developing heart disease is 2.6 mmol/L (100 mg/dL) or less.

High Blood Pressure

Blood pressure refers to the force that blood exerts on the inner walls of the blood vessels as it flows through them. Blood pressure is measured by two numbers: systolic pressure (increased pressure created as your heart muscle contracts) and diastolic (decreased pressure created as your heart muscle relaxes). Up to 27 percent of people with psoriasis have high blood pressure, which is at least 140 mmHg systolic and 90 mmHg diastolic (written 140/90); normal blood pressure is 120/80 or lower.

High Insulin Levels

Insulin is a hormone (a chemical messenger in the body) that helps deliver sugar into the cells so they can use it for fuel. When insulin levels are high, it usually means that the cells aren't responding well to insulin and the body is pumping out large amounts of this hormone to try to compensate. Doctors test insulin levels from time to time because when they start to creep up, it could mean that a person is at risk of developing diabetes. It's possible that the inflammation of psoriasis may also contribute to the chances of having elevated insulin.

Diabetes

In diabetes, the blood has too much sugar in it, either because the body isn't producing enough insulin or because the body has stopped responding properly to the insulin that's already there. While only 4.4 percent of the general Canadian population has diabetes, this disease affects 10 to 12 percent of people with psoriasis. Depending on how severe it is, type 2 diabetes (the most common kind) can be controlled by diet and exercise, or by combining healthy lifestyle changes with various drug treatments, including pills and injected insulin.

Digestive Disorders and Psoriasis

The intestines and skin are alike in many ways. They share similar inflammation and immune mechanisms, which means that someone with psoriasis may be more likely to have **celiac disease** or an inflammatory bowel disease.

Celiac disease causes damage in the small intestine when a person eats **gluten** (see page 142). It leads to diarrhea, weight loss and an inability to absorb nutrients.

"Inflammatory bowel disease" is a term used to describe two conditions—Crohn's disease and ulcerative colitis. Both affect the digestive tract, but in different areas. Crohn's disease can cause inflammation anywhere from the mouth all the way to the anus, whereas ulcerative colitis causes ulceration and inflammation only toward the end of the digestive tract, in the colon (the large intestine).

Both Crohn's disease and ulcerative colitis are more common in people with psoriasis than in the general public. In fact, psoriasis is up to seven times more common in people with Crohn's disease.

Symptoms of inflammatory bowel disease usually include abdominal cramps, fever, weight loss and bloody diarrhea.

Fortunately, there are drugs approved for treating both inflammatory bowel disease and psoriasis. For more information about these treatments, see Chapter 7.

What Is Inflammation? [**MORE DETAIL**]

Inflammation is the body's response to injury or infection. During inflammation, chemicals are released that cause swelling, redness, heat and pain—all of which play a role in healing and protecting surrounding tissues. In conditions such as psoriasis, arthritis and inflammatory bowel disease, the body is sending signals that cause inflammation, even though there may not be an injury or infection present.

Arthritis and Psoriasis

Arthritis is a condition that causes inflammation in the joints. About 40 percent of people with psoriasis get a type of arthritis called psoriatic arthritis because, as with inflammatory bowel disease, these two conditions share a common inflammatory mechanism. In fact, everyone with psoriasis may have some degree of joint inflammation, but only 30 to 50 percent of them develop chronic signs and symptoms of psoriatic arthritis. Genetics probably influence whether psoriasis will lead to serious joint disease, but it's still impossible to predict who will be affected.

Although psoriatic arthritis typically makes an appearance after psoriasis skin symptoms have already developed, it can show up

! [**KEY POINT**]

It's important to get diagnosed as early as possible if you have psoriatic arthritis because the less joint damage you have, the better your medicine will work.

around the same time, or, as is often the case with children, before the skin lesions. Experts aren't sure why, but younger women seem to get the worst cases of psoriatic arthritis. Most people develop this condition between the ages of 20 and 50.

The good news is that it may be possible to treat both psoriasis and psoriatic arthritis with a single drug (see Chapter 7), so be sure to tell your doctor if you have symptoms such as "creakiness" or stiffness in the morning, swelling or pain in your fingers or toes, or pain in your lower back.

What Joints and Tissues Can Be Affected?

Psoriatic arthritis can occur in many or very few joints, usually in the hands, wrists, neck, back, knees, ankles and/or feet. It can lead to joint swelling and deformity, and sometimes to inflammation of other tissues, like the sclera and iris (parts of the eye) or the urethra (the tube that urine passes through). The area around the tendons, called the tendon sheath, can also become inflamed; this condition is called tendonitis.

Sometimes ligaments can swell, but the truest **sign** of psoriatic arthritis is enthesitis, or inflammation that occurs where the tendons insert into the bone. While the bones themselves don't become inflamed, the enthesitis or inflammation around the joints can cause a condition called focal bone destruction. This condition leads to small cysts developing in the bones.

"In my early and late 30s, my arthritic symptoms were so bad that it was 'can I get out of bed?' kind of bad. It was really pretty grisly. Up until that time I had been doing a lot of sporty active things, and I had to give those up."

DAVID

In very severe cases, the joints can totally disintegrate, leading to "telescopic" joints that aren't usually painful but are unable to move properly.

Figure 3.1 Areas of the body most commonly affected by psoriatic arthritis.

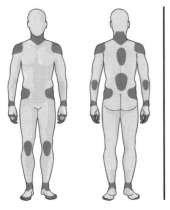

Other Types of Arthritis

A couple of arthritic diseases can be mistaken for psoriatic arthritis and can occur at the same time as psoriatic arthritis:

- Osteoarthritis is very common and is caused by the wear and tear that joints endure in everyday life. In osteoarthritis, joints lose their cushioning and lubrication as cartilage thins.
- Gout is a result of a buildup of uric acid crystals in joints, causing the joints to be tender, red and swollen. This condition is more common in people with psoriasis because their fast rate of skin growth leads to increased uric acid levels.

! [KEY POINT]

It's important to take the other conditions that travel with psoriasis (called **comorbidities**) as seriously as your psoriasis—they won't just disappear on their own or once your psoriasis is under control. So be sure to tell your doctor about any symptoms you are struggling with, even ones that aren't skin problems at all.

Chapter 4

tests and measurements

What Happens in This Chapter
- The steps to diagnosing psoriasis
- Medical tests you might experience
- Other conditions that are sometimes confused
  with psoriasis

*In order to treat your condition, you have to be diagnosed properly. Your doctor
will use several tests and measurements to figure out if you have psoriasis or
another condition, such as eczema, candidiasis or dandruff.*

Introduction

Until now you've probably been dealing with a host of uncomfortable symptoms and it's finally time to figure out exactly what's going on. An accurate diagnosis is always important for getting your condition under control. We encourage you to allow your doctor to conduct any necessary tests and to be honest with him or her when answering questions about your symptoms.

Read Chapter 6 to find out how to make the most of your visits to the doctor.

Diagnosing Psoriasis

Although there is no single test or measurement for diagnosing psoriasis, your doctor will follow a series of diagnostic steps to help identify the condition:

- **Step 1:** Your doctor will ask you questions about your symptoms and health history.
- **Step 2:** Your doctor will examine your skin, scalp and nails for signs of psoriasis.
- **Step 3:** If your diagnosis still isn't clear after Steps 1 and 2, your doctor could perform a skin biopsy, do a joint aspiration test, take an X-ray, ask you to fill out a psoriatic arthritis survey, measure some of your vital signs and/or test your blood.

More About Step 1: Questions You Might Be Asked

Knowing more details about your symptoms, personal health history and family health history will help your doctor decide whether or not you have psoriasis. Common questions you might be asked include:

- What are your symptoms?
- What changes have you noticed in your skin?
- Where on your body have you noticed these skin changes?

- How long have you had these symptoms?
- Do your symptoms come and go at certain times of the year, or do they get worse or better under certain circumstances?
- Do you have any joint pain, swelling or tenderness?
- Have you noticed any changes to your fingernails or toenails?
- Have you had any changes in your bowel function?
- Is there a family history of these types of symptoms or of psoriasis? If so, who in your family was affected?
- Have you already received treatment for any of your symptoms? If so, what were these treatments and were they effective?

Help Yourself to Less Embarrassment   [SELF-HELP]

Although you might feel awkward talking about your symptoms, especially if they're on or near your genitals, remember that your doctor has seen lots of different skin conditions—and on every part of the body. What seems unusual and embarrassing to you is routine for your doctor.

More About Step 2: The Physical Examination

Once you have finished answering questions about your symptoms and health history, you'll be asked to get undressed so that your doctor can examine you. Your doctor will look carefully at:

- Your skin, including your scalp, to identify all the areas where you have skin changes and to determine what kind of psoriasis you might have

- Your fingernails, for signs of pitting (small depressions in the nail plate), lifting of the nail from the nail bed (onycholysis), dead skin accumulating under the nail and small reddish patches under the nail (salmon spots) where psoriasis may be developing
- Your joints, for signs of swelling or tenderness, which could indicate that you have psoriatic arthritis (see page 30)

More About Step 3: Other Possible Tests

Because psoriasis can sometimes seem like other diseases, a review of your health status and a physical examination may not provide your doctor with all the answers he or she needs. In that case, your doctor will have to conduct one or more additional tests to figure out exactly what condition you have.

Skin Biopsy

If your disease is more difficult to diagnose, your doctor might perform a skin biopsy. A biopsy is a simple procedure that lasts only a few minutes and involves removing a sample of your skin so it can be examined under a microscope by a pathologist (a doctor who is specially trained to identify different kinds of diseases). The pathologist will look for certain features in your skin that will help clarify your diagnosis. For more information on what happens during a skin biopsy, see the More Detail box on page 37.

Skin Biopsy Procedure

[**MORE DETAIL**]

Sometimes a skin biopsy is done to check whether you have another condition that can look like psoriasis, such as chronic irritation, long-standing fungal infections and mycosis fungoides (see Is it Really Psoriasis? Other Conditions You Could Have on pages 41 and 44). Having a skin biopsy involves these steps:

- Your doctor may begin by sterilizing the area of skin to be removed with a cotton pad soaked in alcohol. This will feel cool and might sting a bit if your skin is covered by open lesions.
- A small patch of your skin will then be numbed by a needle containing a local anesthetic; this will pinch and sting for a few seconds.
- Once your skin is numbed, or "frozen," your doctor will use an instrument called a punch to remove a 3 to 4 millimeter round patch of skin.
- Your doctor might use a suture—a stitch made by a medical-style needle and thread—to close the wound created by the punch.

X-ray

Your doctor may send you for an X-ray if he or she suspects that you have psoriatic arthritis or another type of arthritis (see page 32). An X-ray will show whether or not you have internal damage to the joints in your hands, wrists, neck, back, knees, ankles and/or feet— areas that are commonly affected by psoriatic arthritis. An X-ray can also show how widespread your arthritis might be.

Sometimes an X-ray is the only way to diagnose psoriatic arthritis, because people with this disease can experience little or no pain. Even if the pain is minimal, there can still be substantial damage to the joint. However, be aware that not all radiologists are experts at detecting the subtle differences between psoriatic arthritis and other arthritic conditions. Make sure your radiologist is familiar with diagnosing psoriatic arthritis, and don't be afraid to ask for a second opinion if you feel you want one.

ToPAS

If your doctor thinks you could have psoriatic arthritis, you may also be asked to fill out a survey called the **Toronto Psoriatic Arthritis Screen (ToPAS)**, designed by Dafna Gladman, a Toronto physician. The ToPAS consists of 14 questions that ask you about your ethnic background, family history of psoriasis and psoriatic arthritis, and personal history of skin rashes, joint pain and other symptoms related to psoriatic arthritis.

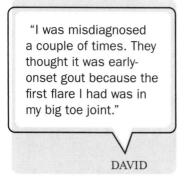

"I was misdiagnosed a couple of times. They thought it was early-onset gout because the first flare I had was in my big toe joint."

DAVID

Joint Aspiration

Another test your doctor may conduct if you are showing signs of arthritis is joint aspiration (see More Detail box on page 39). If that's the case, he or she will use a syringe to take a sample of fluid from an affected joint to look for infection, white blood cells and a type of crystal found in gout (a very painful form of arthritis—see page 32). If any of these signs are present in your joint fluid, you may have something other than psoriatic arthritis.

Joint Aspiration ... Easy as 1, 2, 3 [**MORE DETAIL**]

Getting a joint aspiration test may sound scary, but it's really quite straightforward.

1. Your doctor will start by sterilizing the area of your skin where the needle will enter with betadine, an antiseptic solution.
2. A small needle containing anesthetic will be inserted into your skin to numb, or freeze, the area. This might burn or sting a bit, but the discomfort won't last long because the anesthetic starts to work as soon as it's injected.
3. A larger needle will be inserted into the same area to withdraw fluid from your joint. This part of the procedure shouldn't hurt thanks to the anesthetic, but you might feel some pain if the needle accidentally comes in contact with your bone or cartilage.

Blood and Vital Sign Tests

Your doctor may perform other tests to see whether you have psoriasis comorbidities (see Chapter 3) or other conditions that are unrelated to psoriasis, such as lupus, whose symptoms are similar to those of psoriatic arthritis (see page 43). Blood tests can reveal whether your blood sugar is high, you have inflammation in your body or you test positive for rheumatoid arthritis instead of psoriatic arthritis. Checking your blood pressure allows your doctor to see whether you are showing signs of cardiovascular disease (see Chapter 3), which often occurs along with psoriasis.

Is It Really Psoriasis? Other Conditions You Could Have

Several conditions can be mistaken for psoriasis or can occur at the same time as psoriasis:

- Eczema
- Fungal infections
- Candidiasis (a type of yeast infection)
- Seborrheic dermatitis (dandruff)
- Lupus
- Reactive erythema
- Mycosis fungoides

Eczema

Eczema (pronounced egg-ZEE-mah or EGG-zih-mah), or atopic dermatitis, is a skin condition that can look similar to psoriasis, especially if it has been present for many years or appears thickly on the hands and feet. But there are several key differences between these diseases.

> **!** [**KEY POINT**]
>
> **Eczema** tends to be wet and oozing and easily infected by bacteria, whereas psoriasis plaques are dry and rarely get infected.

Eczema is always extremely itchy and usually appears in the creases of the forearms and behind the knees. Although psoriasis can be itchy, it can be much less itchy than eczema or not itchy at all, and it usually appears on the elbows, knees and scalp in a symmetrical pattern.

Eczema is often accompanied by asthma, as well as seasonal and/or food allergies (the combination of asthma, allergies and eczema is sometimes called the "atopic triad"). In contrast, psoriasis is often accompanied by conditions such as arthritis, cardiovascular disease, depression and inflammatory bowel disease, instead of asthma.

Eczema also gets infected by bacteria easily and is wet and oozing when it first appears. Eczema has no well-defined border separating it from normal skin and commonly has skin cracks. Psoriasis, on the other hand, rarely gets infected, even when the skin is cracked or open. In addition, it has dry, as opposed to wet, lesions with well-defined borders and thick silvery scales, as well as possible nail changes.

Eczema usually appears in childhood, especially in children under 2 years of age, and often clears by the age of 8 or 10. Psoriasis tends to appear in adulthood, although there may be hints earlier (e.g., psoriatic diaper rash in infants or guttate psoriasis in school-aged children).

Fungal Infections

A fungal skin infection known as **ringworm** can resemble psoriasis, thanks to the raised, red, scaly lesions that it can cause on the scalp, body, hands or feet, as well as its tendency to affect the nails. However, there are several ways to tell the two conditions apart.

Ringworm appears in an asymmetrical pattern, whereas psoriasis takes on a symmetrical pattern. Also, ringworm scales aren't silvery like psoriasis scales and they don't appear in the centre of the affected skin—thus "ringworm." Finally, ringworm will test positive for fungus, whereas psoriasis won't. A simple skin scraping or nail clippings can help your doctor determine whether your symptoms are the result of a fungal infection.

Candidiasis

Candidiasis is a type of yeast that can sometimes overgrow in the body, causing an infection. Candida of the skin often looks like red patches surrounded by small pustules. This type of infection is not very common on the genitals, whereas psoriasis on the genitals is quite common. So when candidiasis occurs under the breasts, on the penis or in other body folds, it can easily be mistaken for psoriasis. A simple skin scraping examined under a microscope will help your doctor tell what condition you actually have.

Seborrheic Dermatitis

Most of us think of seborrheic dermatitis, or dandruff, as occurring only in the scalp, but it can also develop on the face. When that happens, it's hard even for experts to tell it apart from facial psoriasis. One clue is whether certain kinds of fungi are found in the irritated part of the skin; if so, it could indicate seborrheic dermatitis rather than psoriasis. Your doctor may want to take a swab of the skin on your face to look into this possibility.

Lupus

Lupus is a chronic disease that causes inflammation in many parts of the body and affects about 50,000 Canadians. Lupus—especially a form of the disease called discoid lupus—can sometimes be confused with psoriasis because its possible symptoms include a red, scaly rash on the body, a red rash that covers the upper cheeks and bridge of the nose, and joint pain and swelling. Your doctor can order blood tests to find out whether you have psoriasis or lupus.

Figure 4.1 Lupus—This is sometimes mistaken for psoriasis

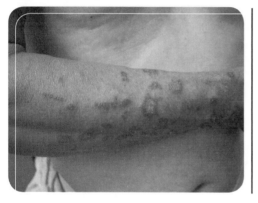

Reactive Erythema

Reactive erythema (pronounced ar-uh-THEE-ma) is redness of the skin that is usually a sign of inflammation or infection. It can sometimes be mistaken for psoriasis.

Mycosis Fungoides

Mycosis fungoides (pronounced my-KO-sis fun-GOY-deez) is a type of cancer called non-Hodgkin's lymphoma that appears on the skin. It is relatively common and usually benign. It often looks like patches of psoriasis and can appear in the same areas as psoriasis, mostly on the buttocks, trunk and thighs.

Figure 4.2 Mycosis fungoides—Another condition that is confused with psoriasis

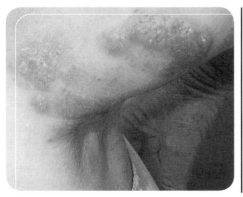

Chapter 5

preparing for your psoriasis journey

What Happens in This Chapter
- Emotions you might experience when you're first diagnosed
- General questions to ask your doctor
- The importance of sharing
- How to navigate the healthcare system

Once you're diagnosed with psoriasis, you will probably experience lots of different feelings—all of which are normal. Your journey ahead may seem overwhelming, but building a support network and learning how to navigate the healthcare system will go a long way toward easing your stress.

You Have Psoriasis—Now What?

When you are first diagnosed with psoriasis, it's normal to experience a whole range of emotions. You might feel relieved because you now have a definite diagnosis, or scared and upset about what your future holds. It's common to feel angry about the "injustice" of your fate and sad that your life isn't what you had hoped. You might even deny that your diagnosis is true.

Most people who are newly diagnosed with psoriasis are concerned that their disease will be with them for life. There are no guarantees about how your condition will develop. You should know that extensive psoriasis is rare and you will probably have limited psoriasis that slowly spreads over time. You may also have many areas of psoriasis that come and go, or a few areas that persist for years or decades. If you get guttate psoriasis, it may clear up within a few months.

Any and all of these concerns and feelings are to be expected when you are told you have a chronic (long-term) disease. But it is important to remember that you're not alone. There are hundreds of thousands of other Canadians with psoriasis who live productive, fulfilling lives—and so can you.

Take some time to let your diagnosis sink in, and make sure all of your questions about it are answered (see Questions for Your Doctor on page 48). There are some things you can do immediately to help yourself—these are outlined in Chapter 8. To minimize itch, cracks and fissures, see Reducing Physical Discomfort on pages 114 to 115. You may also be thinking about emotional and physical challenges; see pages 153 to 169 for some thoughts on overcoming them.

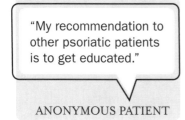

"My recommendation to other psoriatic patients is to get educated."

ANONYMOUS PATIENT

Then you might want to start finding people to give you emotional support (see Forming a Support Network on page 160). We also recommend becoming informed about the healthcare system so you'll be able to better advocate for yourself (see Navigating the Healthcare System on page 50).

Your next step should be to work with your doctor, family and friends so that you can get a treatment plan that will help control your psoriasis and fit with your lifestyle. You can find out about different psoriasis treatment options in Chapter 7.

This is your chance to take control of your health and your life.

Stress Relief!   [SELF-HELP]

If you're feeling overwhelmed by your psoriasis diagnosis, here are a few suggestions to help you deal with your emotions. For more information on how to improve your mood, see Chapters 8 and 11.

• Talk to friends and family, members of a support group or a mental health professional.

• Write down some of your feelings in a journal, including things you're grateful for.

• Have some fun. Laughing can help you feel less stressed (see page 136).

• Talk to your doctor. Often he or she can relieve many of your fears.

• Meditate or do relaxation exercises (see page 165).

• Go for a walk or any kind of workout. The chemicals released when you exercise help you feel calmer (see page 167).

Questions for Your Doctor

When it comes to your health, don't be afraid to speak up. It can sometimes be hard to ask your doctor questions, but remember, it's your body and you have a right to help make decisions about your treatment and fully understand your condition and your options.

Here is a list of questions you might want to ask your doctor to make sure you get all the information you need before going ahead with treatment:

- What kind of psoriasis do I have?
- How many people have you treated with my condition?
- How common is my type of psoriasis, and how easy or hard is it to get under control?
- How is my condition most commonly treated? How long does it usually take to get under control?
- What are my treatment options, including alternative treatments?
- What are the benefits and drawbacks of these treatments?
- What can trigger a flare?
- What kinds of things can I do for fast relief if I suddenly flare?
- Is there anything I should avoid doing (e.g., exercise)?
- What should my daily skin care routine include?
- How often should I come for checkups?
- What types of changes in my condition are considered an emergency? How should I handle an emergency?
- How should I handle a non-emergency injury to my skin (e.g., cuts and scrapes)?
- What other kinds non-skin-related symptoms should I be looking out for? If they appear, should I contact you immediately or wait until our next appointment?
- How do I get in touch with a support group?

The Importance of Sharing

Having sympathetic people around to help you through a crisis and share your fears and concerns with is what makes hard times bearable. In fact, studies confirm that having support over the course of an illness can lead to better and faster healing and an easier time handling the psychological impact of a disease (see page 119).

There are many places you can go for support throughout your psoriasis journey—a professional counselor, your doctors, a patient support group, your friends and family.

If you are nervous talking about your feelings or embarrassed about sharing your experiences, there are other ways to express your frustrations and work through some of your emotions. Journaling, meditating or drawing can all be helpful. You can also join an online support group where you can remain anonymous.

"I think it would have been very helpful to have been able to share experiences with other people who were experiencing similar things and find out what their coping mechanisms might have been—I felt kind of isolated."

DAVID

For more on building a support network, see page 160. For support organizations, see the Resources section in this book.

Navigating the Healthcare System

Fortunately, Canada has a good healthcare system that is available to support you through your psoriasis treatment. It provides everything from free visits to the doctor to special drug benefit plans. However, many Canadians are unaware of all that our system has to offer. Understanding how the system works and what kinds of services it provides can help you get the best possible treatment.

To begin with, our federal government funds each province's healthcare plan through **Medicare**, a program designed to ensure that all Canadians have free access to necessary medical services. Of course, what each person considers necessary and what the government considers necessary are sometimes quite different! For example, someone with psoriasis would probably consider drug coverage necessary, but the government does not.

Nevertheless, there are a few government health benefit programs that provide medications and services free of charge for certain individuals, such as Aboriginal peoples, veterans, members of the military and RCMP, federal inmates and people over age 65 (keep in mind that each program covers different sets of drugs). Some of these benefits are federal (i.e., they apply to all Canadians); some are provincial. Benefits vary from province to province and territory to territory—from free drugs to free medical equipment. You might be surprised at the types of support you're entitled to. To find out more about what your province or territory offers, visit the Resources section in this book.

Whom to Call First

Your family doctor is your central point of contact for all your health issues. If you have a new symptom or think you might need a referral to a specialist (see More Detail box on page 52), your family doctor is the first healthcare professional you should call. Once you have established contact with a specialist physician, you are sometimes allowed to make an appointment directly with that specialist. But the policy in each office regarding new appointments is different.

If you need medical help and you don't have a family doctor, or your specialist is far away, you can go to a walk-in clinic or emergency room. Canadians who live in very remote areas may be eligible for grants that cover the cost of traveling long distances to see a doctor (e.g., the Northern Health Travel Grant Program for residents of Ontario). Be sure to ask your nearest health center for details on these types of programs.

Specialist Physician Referrals

You may go your entire life dealing with one doctor—your family physician—or you may end up getting referred to one or more specialist physicians. These specialists include dermatologists (who deal with skin), rheumatologists (who deal with joints), gastroenterologists (who deal with the digestive system), psychiatrists (who deal with emotional issues) and cardiologists (who deal with the heart). Family doctors usually make referrals when:

- Your disease is more severe, based on the extent of your psoriasis and the amount of your distress
- Your psoriasis occurs in areas that are particularly difficult to treat, such as the scalp, palms of your hands and soles of your feet
- You require more in-depth counseling that falls outside the scope of a family practice
- Your diagnosis is unclear
- There is a need for help in developing an appropriate treatment
- You don't respond to or have stopped responding to therapy
- Your face, scalp, hands, feet or areas around and including your genitals are affected
- You have a more complicated type of psoriasis, such as pustular or erythrodermic psoriasis
- You have one or more comorbidities (see Chapter 3), such as cardiovascular disease, depression, inflammatory bowel disease or arthritis
- You request a referral

Be aware that it can take a long time (weeks to months) to get your first appointment with a specialist physician. However, once you establish contact, it becomes much quicker and easier to book an appointment.

Your physician will tell you whom he or she would prefer you contact if your psoriasis becomes worse or you develop a new symptom. If your doctor doesn't mention this, be sure to ask about it. Some might want you to pay your family doctor a visit first, while others might want you to contact your specialist physician directly. Talk to your doctors about developing a plan of action that will work for all of you.

Finding a Doctor Who Fits

Just like the chemistry can be "off" when you go on a date, patients and doctors don't always "click." The personality, style and interests of your healthcare providers can sometimes clash with yours. Some doctors are more direct, while others take a subtler approach. Some doctors will prefer to let you make up your own mind about therapies rather than directing you to a specific treatment. Some doctors are very interested in research, while others are not.

The bottom line is, if you don't feel comfortable with the diagnosis you've been given or don't like working with one or more of the doctors you've seen, don't be afraid to seek out another family doctor or ask for a referral to a different specialist. It will be much easier to get your condition under control if you and your doctors get along.

It may also be worth doing a little homework if you need a specialist. Some dermatologists focus more on cosmetics and are less likely to be interested in or have the time to treat psoriasis, while others are more focused on treating skin cancer or other conditions. Ask around.

Drug Benefits

One of the main issues that people with psoriasis face is the cost of drug therapies. While some private plans will pay for pharmaceutical treatments, a few of the more powerful drugs are very expensive and aren't always covered by private insurance programs. You may qualify for financial assistance from the government if you have additional challenges (see Services for Canadians with Additional Challenges below) or be eligible to join a **clinical trial**.

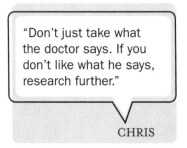

"Don't just take what the doctor says. If you don't like what he says, research further."

CHRIS

Chapter 7 has more information on how to get funding for your medication if the government doesn't cover you (see page 98).

Services for Canadians With Additional Challenges

The government offers special assistance to certain groups of people who may have challenges in addition to their psoriasis. These groups include veterans, people over age 65, people with permanent disabilities, recent immigrants, students, parents, low-income earners, individuals in remote locations and Aboriginal peoples.

What these groups are entitled to differs from province to province and territory to territory, but there are some federal programs available across Canada. These include Non-Insured Health Benefits (NIHB) for First Nations and Inuit, and Communities Achieving Responsive Services (CARS) for people living in rural, remote or northern Canada. You'll find contact information for these types of programs in the Resources section of this book.

What Does the Future Hold?

The wonderful thing about the future is that no one knows what it holds—of course, that's also what can make it scary. You cannot predict the course your disease will take. The next few weeks, months and years will likely be filled with both frustration and joy. The best you can do is hope for the best, plan for the worst and live in the present.

Make the most of each good day and be prepared to face the bad days knowing that they will eventually give way to happy times. A psoriasis diagnosis does not mean that you'll never enjoy yourself again. It's simply one of the many bumps in the road you will face as you go through life. We all have our own list of challenges to overcome, and one of yours happens to be psoriasis.

"It's a tough thing to get through. But if you stay tough and hang tough and have the right frame of mind, you can get through it."

MARGIE

Chapter 6

making the most of visiting your doctor

What Happens in This Chapter
- How to prepare for your visit and what to ask
- Health professionals you might encounter

Going to the doctor can feel overwhelming, but if you know what to expect and come prepared, your visits will be productive and your physician and his or her team will be able to give you the help you need. This chapter gives you tips and tricks for getting the most out of your visits with the healthcare professionals you might encounter.

How to Prepare for Visits

Whether you have an appointment with your family doctor, a dermatologist or a dietitian, you can do a few things ahead of time to make your visit run smoothly.

What to Bring

It's important that the medical professionals you're dealing with have all of the information about your health so they can come up with the best possible treatment plan for you. When you come to your doctor's office, be sure to bring:

- A list of all your prescription medications and nutrition supplements
- Your complete medical history (e.g., major surgeries, major childhood illnesses, vaccinations received, history of smoking and alcohol consumption, ongoing infections such as hepatitis or HIV), including your family's medical history (e.g., a list of family members who had a heart attack or stroke before age 60, the number of parents and siblings with psoriasis)
- A list of the questions you want to ask your doctor (see pages 48, 63 and 190)
- A list of answers to the most common questions doctors ask (see What You Will Be Asked on page 58).

…or and his or her staff are there to help you in any way
…However, keep in mind that they are very busy, so knowing
…ask what can go a long way toward making your visits as
…t as possible—for you and your healthcare team. Here are a
…'s and don'ts:

	Don't
…ask the receptionist about …pointments and whether your lab …sults are in	Don't ask the receptionist about your symptoms or medications
…o ask your doctor any questions you might have about your condition, including symptoms, treatment options and side effects	Don't hesitate to ask the receptionist about booking your next appointment
Do talk to your doctor about making sure you have enough medication until your next appointment	Don't ask the receptionist to cancel an appointment at the last minute— be sure that you honour the office's cancellation policy

What You Will Be Asked

Another way to get the most out of visiting your doctor is to be prepared for what he or she might ask you. Thinking about your answers in advance will allow you to give accurate and complete information, which can help your doctor create a more effective treatment plan for you.

1. *How long have you had psoriasis?* If your psoriasis has developed more recently (i.e., within several months), it is often more responsive to treatment.

2. *Do you have psoriatic arthritis or joint disease related to psoriasis?* Some treatments are effective at treating both the skin and joints, while some are better for treating either joints or skin (e.g., creams won't help joint disease).

3. *How extensive is your psoriasis?* If your psoriasis covers less than a few palms' worth of skin on your body, it can usually be treated with creams, whereas several palms of psoriasis scattered over different areas of your body will be difficult to treat topically.

4. *How much does the psoriasis bother you?* If you're not bothered by your psoriasis, your doctor can probably skip the more "aggressive" therapies. If your psoriasis bothers you a lot, you and your doctor can talk about more powerful treatment options.

5. *Do any of your family members have psoriasis?*

6. *Do any of your family members have multiple sclerosis?*

7. *Where were you born?* This question is important in identifying your risk of being exposed to tuberculosis.

8. *What other treatments have you tried for your psoriasis?*

If you're seeing a nutritionist or dietitian, you might also be asked to fill out a food diary that tracks everything you've eaten over several days.

Who Will Be in the Office?

Getting to know the health professionals you might encounter when you go to the doctor is another important step to getting the most out of your treatment. Here is a rundown of all of the potential people on your support team and their roles:

Dermatologist: A dermatologist is a medical doctor who specializes in treating diseases of the skin, nails and hair. You may be referred to a dermatologist if you and your family doctor are having trouble getting your psoriasis under control.

Endocrinologist: An endocrinologist is a medical doctor who specializes in treating diseases that affect the endocrine, or hormonal, system. If you have diabetes, you may be sent to see an endocrinologist.

Family doctor: Your family doctor is your home base and first line of contact if you experience any changes in your health status. Your family doctor can treat you directly or refer you to other specialist physicians, such as a dermatologist or psychiatrist.

Holistic nutritionist: A holistic nutritionist is a professional who can help you plan meals and choose healthy foods. Nutritionists don't undergo as many years of schooling as registered dietitians, but they are trained to make individualized suggestions for improving your health that take into account your body, mind and spirit.

Naturopathic doctor: A naturopathic doctor is an alternative healthcare practitioner who has undergone as many years of schooling as a regular medical doctor, but who has been trained in alternative modalities, such as homeopathy, nutrition and herbalism. Naturopaths can't give you pharmaceutical drugs, but they can recommend nutritional supplements and other non-prescription treatments.

Psychiatrist: A psychiatrist is a medical doctor who specializes in treating people with mental health problems, such as depression and anxiety. Psychiatrists can recommend stress reduction techniques and give you guidance on how to overcome emotional roadblocks. They can also prescribe medication. If you are finding it hard to deal with the social and emotional challenges of your psoriasis, you can ask your family doctor for a referral to a psychiatrist.

Psychologist: A psychologist usually has a PhD in psychology and is trained to help people who are suffering from mental health problems, such as depression and anxiety. Psychologists can recommend stress reduction techniques and give you guidance on how to overcome emotional roadblocks, but they can't prescribe medication. If you are finding it hard to deal with the psychological challenges of your psoriasis, you can consult a psychologist.

Receptionist: The receptionist is the person you'll talk to on the phone when you call your doctor's office, and he or she will be the first to greet you when you arrive for an appointment. Receptionists are responsible for the administration of the office, relaying messages from your doctor and booking appointments.

Registered dietitian: A registered dietitian often works closely with medical professionals to ensure that your diet is healthy and complements your other treatments. A dietitian has a university degree in the field of nutrition, but is not trained in the same sorts of alternative modalities as a holistic nutritionist.

Registered nurse: A registered nurse assists doctors and acts as a patient advocate. Nurses might ask you questions before you see a physician, and they will often perform tests, such as taking your blood or checking your blood pressure.

Rheumatologist: A rheumatologist is a medical doctor who has specialized training in treating diseases of the joints, muscles and bones. You might see a rheumatologist if you have psoriatic arthritis.

Chapter 7

which treatment is right for you?

What Happens in This Chapter
- Treatment-related questions to ask your doctor
- Lifestyle factors that can influence your treatment
- Overview of prescription and non-prescription topical treatments, light therapy, systemic treatments and combination therapies
- How to know whether your treatment is working
- Funding your treatment
- A quick reference guide to therapies

There are many psoriasis treatments available. The therapies you end up using will depend on how severe your condition is and your lifestyle. Unless your psoriasis is very severe, your doctor will probably start you on a topical medication that you apply directly to your skin. If topical treatments don't work, there are lots of other options, such as light therapy, combination therapies and systemic drugs that you take as a pill, by injection or by infusion. Although some treatments can be quite expensive, you may be able to get financial help through the government or drug companies.

Introduction

There are now more therapies than ever to effectively control your psoriasis, but the type of treatment your doctor recommends for you will depend on what kind of psoriasis you have, its location and how severe it is. Your treatment will also depend on what medications react best with you, other medications you may be taking, your drug plan and your lifestyle.

Regardless of which therapy you're on, you will most likely be treated at home—because we now have a better understanding of psoriasis and better therapies, hospitalizing someone for psoriasis is a thing of the past. The only time you could end up in the hospital is if your psoriasis gets so bad that your life is in danger, such as with erythrodermic psoriasis (see page 18). However, a life-threatening case of psoriasis is extremely rare. In all likelihood, your psoriasis will never cause you to spend a night in the hospital.

Although individual doctors may take slightly different approaches with each of their psoriasis patients, we've outlined some general guidelines for treating this condition. For more information about alternative and complementary treatment options, and how to eat well and stay healthy, read Chapters 9 and 10.

Questions for Your Doctor

To help you understand which treatment is right for you, it is important that you get as much information as possible about all your options. Here are some questions that you might want to ask your doctor:

- What treatments are most appropriate for my type of psoriasis?
- How successful are they? How long do they usually take to work?

- If these treatments don't work, what are my other options?
- How might these treatments affect my lifestyle?
- Which drugs, herbs and supplements that I'm already on might interact with my psoriasis medication?
- Could any foods interact with my psoriasis medication?
- What are the risks or potential side effects of the psoriasis treatments you're considering for me?
- Will the side effects eventually go away? If so, how long will that take?
- How much will my treatment cost?
- Are there any clinical trials that I can join?

Lifestyle and Treatment Choice: They Go Hand in Hand

Many lifestyle factors affect what kind of treatment your doctor chooses for you:

- **Occupation:** If you travel a lot for work or can't leave your workplace in the middle of the day, you'll need treatments that are portable. Some treatments, such as phototherapy, might not be an option for you. Also, taking medications on trips can be complicated due to airport security, customs and storage. It's important to keep drugs from getting too cold or too hot, and if you're taking injections, you'll need to get a letter of explanation from your dermatologist to get your medication past airport security, especially when crossing an international border.

- **Location:** If you live far away from medical facilities, you may have trouble getting to a clinic where certain drugs are administered by intravenous infusion. However, most infusions are given every few weeks, and some people find it far more convenient to spend 2 or 3 hours every 6 to 8 weeks getting their treatment. Location is also an issue with ultraviolet light treatment, since few treatment facilities exist and you may have to travel a long distance to receive your therapy.

- **Medical coverage**: It's unfortunate that the amount of medical coverage has to influence access to treatment. The reality is, though, if you don't have private insurance, don't qualify for government drug benefits (see page 50) and aren't eligible for a clinical trial (see page 98), some of the more expensive treatment options may be out of reach.
- **Health status**: If you have other health issues and are taking medications that interact with psoriasis drugs, your psoriasis treatment might be limited. For example, if you are overweight or have psoriatic arthritis, hypertension, high cholesterol, or poor liver or kidney function, there are fewer medications available to control your psoriasis.
- **Life goals**: Life plans can sometimes get in the way of psoriasis treatment. For example, if you are pregnant (or if you plan to get pregnant soon) some **oral treatments** won't be appropriate for you. If you are traveling to a remote location, you may need to make arrangements to store your drugs or get access to medical care.

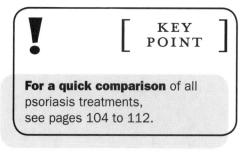

! [**KEY POINT**]

For a quick comparison of all psoriasis treatments, see pages 104 to 112.

Topical Treatments:
The Logical Starting Point

A topical treatment is one that you apply to the outside of your body. Topicals come in various forms, such as a spray, ointment, cream, gel or liquid. If your psoriasis is mild, you will be prescribed topical therapies—they are usually a great treatment starting point. If your psoriasis is more severe, your doctor may ask you to combine topical therapies with other kinds of treatments (see Combination Therapies on page 95) or take systemic drugs (see page 78). For a quick reference to topical treatments, see page 104.

The Do's and Don'ts of Topicals

Applying topicals can be bit more complicated than simply spreading a cream, lotion or ointment on your skin. This section provides a few do's and don'ts to make it easier.

For most areas, you can dab your topical on your psoriasis and then spread it thinly with your fingers. To find out how to apply topicals to trickier areas, keep reading this section. Don't apply your topicals anywhere that your doctor hasn't specifically given you permission to—more sensitive areas of the body can't tolerate certain kinds of medications. It's also important to wash your hands after applying your topical (unless your medication is meant to treat your hands), and always make sure you have enough of your topical to last until your next doctor's appointment (see More Detail box on page 67).

Cream Calculator

It's easy to figure out if you have enough medication to last until your next doctor's appointment if you use the "palm rule." The palm of your hand is about 1 percent of your total body surface, and you'll need 0.5 g of cream or lotion for every palm's worth of area on your body with psoriasis.

For example, suppose you have two "palms" of psoriasis on your arms and two "palms" on your legs. You will use 2 g of cream or ointment with every application and you will need about 60 g in a month, if you're going to use your topical once a day. It takes about 1 g of cream or lotion (about the size of a small pea) to cover your face and about 50 g to cover your whole body.

Figure 7.1 This is what 0.5g of cream looks like

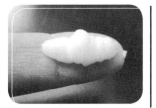

How to Remove and Apply Topicals to Hairy Body Areas

It's important to clean off the last application of your topical before applying the next one. Removing a topical from body parts with lots of hair, such as the scalp or arms, can be tough. To overcome this challenge, simply apply lots of cheap shampoo (the cheapest you can find) *before* you get your hair wet. Work the shampoo into your skin and hair, let it sit for 2 minutes and then rinse it out—it will "dissolve" the gel, lotion or cream. Then you can shampoo normally and be free of residue from your medication.

After you shampoo, you can re-apply your medication. To apply it to you scalp, start by towel drying your hair so it's still damp. Then part your hair, touch the nozzle of the lotion bottle to your skin and spread the drop of medication over your scalp with your fingers. You can test how much of the topical comes out of the bottle at once by applying a drop to the back of your hand; this should leave enough solution to cover most of that area. On your scalp, the same-sized drop will cover about half the area it did on your hand because some of it will be absorbed by your hair (dry hair absorbs more).

How to Apply Topicals to the Ears
If you are using a medicated shampoo, put some of it in your ears at the beginning of your shower or bath and rinse it out at the end. Then dry your ears gently with a paper towel draped over your index finger or, better yet, just let your ears air dry.

If you are applying a cream, lotion or liquid medication to your ears, be sure to keep your fingernails short. Apply a drop of your topical to your index finger and gently rub it into your ear canal. Avoid putting your finger too far in your ears, or you could hurt your eardrum.

And whatever you do, don't use cotton swabs to apply medication to your ears—cotton swabs have the potential to puncture your ear drum. They are also irritating, and your ears will become very itchy within about 2 or 3 days of using them. If you've already started using cotton swabs and are finding it hard to stop, go cold turkey. The itching should go away in under a week.

How to Apply Topicals to the Hands, Feet, Elbows and Knees
A good time to apply ointments to the hands, feet, elbows and knees is right before going to bed. Once your medication is on, put on thin cotton gloves or socks so it won't rub off on your sheets or clothing. You can use an old pair of socks with the toecap cut off to cover your elbows and knees.

How to Apply Topicals to Hard-to-Reach Places
If you can, avoid putting on a topical by yourself if your psoriasis is in a hard-to-see or hard-to-reach area—try asking someone for help. If you live alone and don't have help, ask your doctor for suggestions on how best to apply your medication.

How to Apply Topicals Near the Eyes
Always apply your medication carefully near your eyes, and wash it off gently if you react to it. You can try to apply it again in a day or two if the irritation is mild. If it's more severe, contact your doctor and stop using the cream or lotion altogether. Never allow a topical—even a simple moisturizer—to stay around your eyes if you find it irritating.

Corticosteroids

The most common medications used to relieve mild psoriasis symptoms are topical corticosteroids (also called steroids). They come in the form of lotions, creams, ointments, foams or oils that you rub on your skin. Lotions are most often used for hairy skin or skin folds, and creams are used because they are cosmetically more acceptable. For scalp psoriasis, there are also shampoos.

Steroids are powerful anti-inflammatory drugs that can reduce swelling, pain, itching and redness. There are many different steroids that come in many different strengths. For example, hydrocortisone is the weakest steroid, so it can be used on your face, genitals and skin folds—at least for short periods of time. Betamethasone valerate is much more potent than hydrocortisone, and clobetasol is among the most powerful corticosteroids. Both betamethasone and clobetasol should only be used for a few weeks at a time. It's important to follow your doctor's instructions carefully when using steroids.

> ❗ **[KEY POINT]**
>
> **There are many different** kinds of steroids of many different strengths. You must always follow your doctor's instructions when applying your steroid medication.

Because topical steroids can cause side effects if used too often, your doctor may recommend "pulse-dosing," which involves changing how often and how much of the medication you use every few weeks. For example, you might use your steroid cream twice daily for 2 weeks and then once daily for 2 days of each week for the next 8 weeks. If you find that you need to use your steroid every day, see your dermatologist, because you shouldn't have to apply it often after you've been on it for a couple of weeks.

The most common side effect of steroids is thinning of the skin—also called "atrophy." When the surface of your skin becomes very thin, it may develop wrinkles that look like thin, crumpled paper. If the steroid isn't stopped occasionally, the atrophy can lead to bruising and fragility of the skin, causing it to tear or scratch more easily. Another common side effect of steroids is a skin condition that looks like acne, but isn't. Sometimes a more potent steroid is used to suppress this condition, but this only causes more problems—the best way to get rid of the "acne" is to stop using steroids for 1 or 2 weeks.

Stretch marks, called *striae distensae* or just *striae* (pronounced STREE-ay), can also develop when you use steroids. Although these stretch marks can occur anywhere, they are found more often in areas where the skin is thinnest, such as the groin and armpits. This is a much less common side effect than skin thinning or an acne-like condition, but some people are more sensitive to steroids and can develop stretch marks even when they use the mildest forms of these drugs for short periods of time. Keep in mind that just because you already have stretch marks (and most of us have a few somewhere) doesn't mean that you are more susceptible to developing stretch marks with steroid use.

Doctors will sometimes inject steroids into psoriasis plaques that don't respond well to topical therapy. This approach can be quite effective, but it hasn't been studied very carefully and it probably poses the same risks that doctors worry about with powerful steroid creams and ointments, such as skin thinning and other permanent changes. However, steroid injections can be reasonably safe and helpful for very limited areas of psoriasis and for regions such as the scalp, elbows and knees.

Steroids might not be an option for you if you become allergic to them. One of the signs of an allergic reaction to your steroid is if your psoriasis seems to be getting worse and itchier, rather than better. Testing patches of your skin can help your doctor figure out if you are allergic to the steroid or to a component of the cream that the steroid sits in. Nevertheless, steroids are still a great choice for many people and are sometimes the only treatment that works and is available and affordable.

Vitamin D–Based Medications

Some topical psoriasis treatments take advantage of the healing effects of vitamin D (see More Detail box on page 72). Calcipotriol is a vitamin D-based ointment that is often used with other treatments for psoriasis. If your doctor prescribes calcipotriol (called calcipotriene outside Canada), it will probably be in combination with a steroid drug called betamethasone dipropionate (see page 95), which treats psoriasis much more effectively than when you use calcipotriol alone.

The Vitamin D Connection [MORE DETAIL]

Vitamin D plays many important roles in your body. It allows you to absorb calcium, boosts your immunity, reduces inflammation and helps regulate cell growth. However, excessive amounts of vitamin D can be hazardous, potentially causing nausea, vomiting, reduced appetite, constipation, weakness and weight loss. They can also lead to high levels of calcium in your blood, which can cause confusion and heart rhythm abnormalities. That's why you shouldn't try to self-medicate with very high doses of vitamin D supplements. The risk of side effects is just too great.

If you find that calcipotriol irritates your skin, wash the area where you've applied it with a gentle cleanser and water. Although you may not be able to use this medication again, sometimes a break of a few days between applications will do the trick and you can go back to using calcipotriol with minimal side effects. However, some people find that the irritation occurs every time they use calcipotriol, and they end up trying a different treatment.

Calcipotriol works by slowing skin growth and calming the overactive white blood cells that are misdirected in psoriasis. It can even be effective in getting moderate and severe plaque psoriasis under control, but you can't use it on sensitive areas, such as your face. Apply only as much as you need, and be sure to stop and see your doctor if you develop an irritation or allergic reaction to it.

There is also a new vitamin D-based treatment called calcitriol ointment. Like calcipotriol, calcitriol can help control the overgrowth of your skin cells, but it can be applied to sensitive skin areas (e.g., the face) and you can use it continuously for 1 year.

Tacrolimus and Pimecrolimus

Tacrolimus (Protopic) and pimecrolimus (Elidel) are usually used to treat eczema, but they are sometimes prescribed for psoriasis on the face or in folds where the skin is very thin. Neither works very well on other areas of the body because the skin is too thick.

Tazarotene

Tazarotene is a retinoid, meaning it comes from vitamin A, which is known for its immune-regulating powers and skin-healing properties. Like vitamin D, this cream controls skin growth and reduces inflammation, but it can be very irritating to the skin, even when combined with steroids. If you aren't bothered by this, tazarotene can be quite effective at clearing your plaques.

Non-prescription Topical Treatments

Your doctor will probably encourage you to moisturize your skin daily with emollients, creams, lotions or ointments because they may reduce the amount that your skin flakes, cracks, itches and bleeds. They can also make steroid creams and ointment more effective, so you have to use less of them to get relief for your symptoms. For most people with limited psoriasis (i.e., less than one palm of psoriasis) that is thin (i.e., very little scaling and the affected skin feels very similar to normal skin), a moisturizer is probably all that's needed to keep their condition under control.

Lotions, creams and ointments all have very different moisturizing effects. Lotions are thin and used for skin folds or the scalp because they spread very easily. However, lotions aren't all that moisturizing and might need to be applied six to ten times a day to provide the same moisturizing effect as an ointment. Ointments, such as petroleum jelly, are very thick. They are good moisturizers and may make your medication work better. A cream is somewhere in the middle— thicker and more moisturizing than a lotion, but thinner and less moisturizing than an ointment.

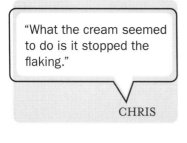

"What the cream seemed to do is it stopped the flaking."

CHRIS

You are free to use almost any kind of moisturizer you like. There are dozens of different products to choose from— literally something for everyone! So experiment until you find one with a texture and smell that you like, and use it regularly. They're great for limited areas of skin, but if more than 5 percent of your body is covered in psoriasis, applying moisturizers might take too much time and effort to apply to be worth it.

Be aware, though, that some moisturizers may have side effects such as irritation or itching. Uncommon problems include allergic reactions (red, thickened, itchy skin), skin irritation and, very rarely, an acne-like eruption, or folliculitis. If your psoriasis seems to get worse when you start using a moisturizer, contact your dermatologist so that he or she can determine whether you're having an allergic reaction or whether your psoriasis has become more severe.

Applying fish oil-based topicals to the skin is another non-prescription treatment that some people with psoriasis turn to because they believe that the anti-inflammatory properties of fish oil will help reduce their discomfort. However, there isn't a lot of research supporting the use of these ointments, and it's possible that the benefit is the same as you would get from a simple moisturizer.

Tar from coal, shale or pitch is also a non-prescription psoriasis therapy. It has been used to treat psoriasis for over a century and is sometimes used alone in low concentrations or in a "treated form" called LCD (*liquor carbolis detergens*).

Tar used to be a popular option for treating mild psoriasis, but it tends to be less effective than other topical medications and has drawbacks, such as its bad smell, potential to irritate the skin, and ability to stain clothes and hair. Some countries have even banned tars because of the theoretical risk of cancer caused by the thousands of chemicals they contain. However, there is no evidence that tar causes cancer when used appropriately. As a result of its many shortcomings, tar isn't recommended as often as it once was, but it remains a common ingredient in everyday products such as medicated shampoos, which don't have a strong odour.

If your skin gets irritated while you're using tar, wash it off with a no-name baby shampoo, which should be applied to your dry skin and then rinsed off gently. Take a break from using the tar, and then try it again in a few days. If you develop an allergic reaction or pustules, wash the tar preparation off and contact your doctor.

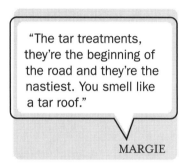

"The tar treatments, they're the beginning of the road and they're the nastiest. You smell like a tar roof."

MARGIE

Light Therapy—An Old Idea Reinvented

Before pharmaceutical treatments existed, people with psoriasis were advised to vacation in warm climates so they could soak up the sun's ultraviolet (UV) rays, which help control skin cell growth and therefore psoriasis.

Nowadays you can go to special clinics to receive regular light therapy treatments. These are safer than sun exposure because the intensity of the rays can be adjusted according to your skin type. For example, if you have very pale skin, your phototherapy technician will reduce the strength of the UV rays so you don't burn. Your doctor might recommend light therapy if you have moderate to severe psoriasis, and it is particularly good for treating guttate psoriasis.

Figure 7.2 A light therapy booth

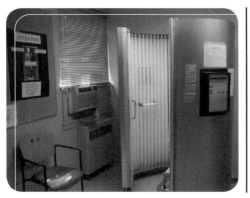

The most commonly prescribed type of light therapy is UVB. If you are exposed to these rays frequently enough (usually three times a week), they can lead to a complete elimination of your psoriasis symptoms. However, there isn't enough research for us to know whether these treatments increase your risk of developing cancer, plus they can be inconvenient because you have to find the time to travel to them. Some doctors have an open-door policy that allows you to come for a treatment whenever it's convenient for you, while others maintain strictly scheduled phototherapy hours.

UVA treatment is another form of phototherapy that can be very successful, even in severe cases of psoriasis. Because UVA is always used in combination with a plant compound called psoralen, you may hear this treatment called by its abbreviation, "**PUVA.**" The psoralen in PUVA makes your skin more sensitive to the effects of the UV light. Psoralen can be taken orally, or you might be asked to add it to your bathwater and soak yourself before being exposed to UVA.

However, PUVA treatment is less appealing than UVB for some people. Bathing with psoralen adds an extra time-consuming step, and oral psoralen can cause stomach upset. Also, if you have a history of receiving PUVA treatments, you may not be allowed to take drugs such as cyclosporine that affect your immune system.

For safety reasons, you shouldn't have more than 200 PUVA sessions over the course of your lifetime. PUVA is also falling out of favor because it's complicated to administer and can raise your risk of developing skin cancer. Whether you get PUVA or UVB therapy, you will need to wear goggles or sunglasses to protect your eyes from ultraviolet light. Phototherapy may also not be the best option for some people, such as anyone:

- With lupus
- With photodermatosis (dermatitis, lupus or hives caused by exposure to ultraviolet light)
- Who gets worse instead of better with phototherapy
- With a history of skin cancer

But it all depends on how easy your psoriasis is to control with other treatments and how much of a risk you're willing to take. Talk to your doctor about whether trying light therapy is right for you.

For a quick reference to phototherapy, see page 106.

"PUVA probably worked better than anything. But the doctor's office was only open certain hours, so I would have to get an extended lunch time, leave work, go home, jump in the bath, soak in the bath for 10 or 15 minutes with [psoralen] dumped in the water, get out, fly down to the doctor's office, get in, get zapped with the lights and get back to work."

CHRIS

Help Yourself to Safer Light Therapy

[SELF-HELP]

Light therapy, or phototherapy, can be an effective way to control your psoriasis, especially if you follow a few simple tips and tricks:

- Don't sit in the sun after you have a phototherapy session.
- Keep your skin moisturized.
- Wear sunscreen *after* your UVB sessions—putting on sunscreen before your treatment will prevent it from working.
- Be consistent when applying moisturizer close to your treatments. A moisturizer will increase the amount of ultraviolet light that gets into your skin, so always apply your moisturizer either before *or* after you get your UVB treatment.

Systemic Treatments: More Help When You Need It

A **systemic treatment** is one that affects the whole body (the whole "system") and is taken orally or injected, rather than rubbed on the skin. Your doctor will usually suggest a systemic therapy if you have a more severe case of psoriasis and will sometimes combine these treatments with phototherapy or topical medications to make them work even better (see Combination Therapies on page 95). For a quick reference to systemic treatments, see page 106.

Acitretin

Like tazarotene (see page 73), acitretin is a retinoid, a drug that comes from vitamin A. Unlike tazarotene, acitretin is taken orally and has more potential side effects than the topical treatment. In addition, this drug is rarely effective when used alone and is usually combined with other treatments (see Combination Therapies on page 95). Other downsides are that acitretin doesn't work well for psoriatic arthritis, and most people find that it takes several weeks before they see an improvement in their skin once they start taking it.

Acitretin is a useful drug for many people with more severe psoriasis, but it causes birth defects, and this effect continues for some years, even after you have stopped it. If you are a woman in your child-bearing years, acitretin may not be for you (see Pregnancy and Acitretin on page 80).

Acitretin's most common side effect is dryness—dry skin, dry eyes and dry lips. Applying moisturizers frequently will help your skin feel normal, smooth and comfortable, and non-medicated eye drops can help your eyes feel better. You can also apply lip balm, particularly one with beeswax, to soothe your chapped or cracked lips.

Stiff joints and sore muscles are also side effects of this drug. If you are exercising or doing physically demanding work, warm up and stretch for 5 to 10 minutes before and 10 minutes after to minimize any achiness. You can also try icing sore joints. You may experience hair loss on acitretin, and your cholesterol may increase. In addition, if you're diabetic, your diabetes may become harder to control.

> **!** **[KEY POINT]**
>
> **It's important** that you avoid drinking alcohol and taking vitamin A supplements while you're on acitretin because they will increase your risk of experiencing dangerous side effects. Alcohol, for example, impairs your body's ability to break down acitretin.

Sometimes going off acitretin for a couple of days will help control its side effects. However, most of the time, the side effects are too great for most people to tolerate at doses that give the best results. Call your doctor if you're finding acitretin's side effects bothersome, so you can figure out next steps together.

Acitretin is safe if you have a history of skin cancer or lymphoma, but a lot of people shouldn't use acitretin. For example, if you have high cholesterol or liver disease, acetretin may not be a good choice for you. Most importantly, women who are pregnant shouldn't use acitretin under any circumstances (see More Detail box below). This means that you should avoid acitretin if you are a woman in your child-bearing years who has difficulty using birth control reliably, or you think you might become pregnant within 3 years.

Pregnancy and Acitretin [**MORE DETAIL**]

Acitretin is **teratogenic**, meaning it can cause a fetus to develop abnormally. That's why you aren't allowed to use this medication if you're a woman of child-bearing age unless you can commit to using birth control during your treatment and for 3 years after your treatment. If you do become pregnant within 3 years of taking acitretin, contact your family doctor, dermatologist and obstetrician immediately—and be prepared that they may recommend an abortion. You also have to wait at least 3 years after stopping your acitretin treatment before donating blood. There is no research on the effects of acitretin on sperm, so there are no official recommendations about whether or not you should stop taking this medication if you are a man who is considering fathering a child.

Cyclosporine

Cyclosporine is a calcineurin inhibitor, a type of drug that affects the immune system. You may recall from Chapter 1 that psoriasis is caused by a misdirected immune system; cyclosporine works by helping to regulate out-of-control white blood cells.

This drug has a long and interesting history. It comes from a fungus called *Tolypocladium inflatum* and was discovered in the 1970s. Cyclosporine was first used in transplant patients because it suppresses the immune system and helps prevent organ rejection. The fact that some of those transplant patients suddenly got their lifelong psoriasis under control was the first hint that psoriasis is connected to the immune system. Today, cyclosporine is used to treat several diseases related to the immune system, such as psoriasis and rheumatoid arthritis, and topical drugs that are related to cyclosporine (e.g., tacrolimus and pimecrolimus) are commonly used in eczema and sometimes in psoriasis.

Cyclosporine can start to relieve psoriatic itching after the first or second dose, with visible skin changes occurring 1 or 2 weeks into treatment. However, it doesn't have much effect on psoriatic arthritis. Cyclosporine comes in the form of a pill that you swallow, usually once or twice a day.

Cyclosporine can affect kidneys, blood pressure and triglyceride levels, so if you have kidney disease, uncontrolled high blood pressure or high cholesterol, this drug may not be for you. You also shouldn't take cyclosporine if you have lymphoma or skin cancer, and although it doesn't appear to cause birth defects, it has been linked to low birth weight.

In addition, you might experience temporary tingling in your fingers, toes, lips and face triggered by temperature changes;

headaches; muscle aches; or stomach upset. To lessen any stomach symptoms, you can try taking cyclosporine on an empty stomach, or with or after meals. Headaches and muscle pain are usually short-lived, but if they persist, your doctor can lower your medication dose. About 10 percent of people who take cyclosporine develop side effects that are bad enough to make them stop treatment. Once you stop treatment, you run the risk of experiencing a rebound or worsening of your psoriasis symptoms, although this should settle down after a few weeks.

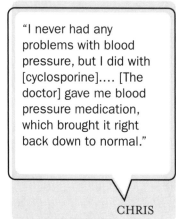

"I never had any problems with blood pressure, but I did with [cyclosporine].... [The doctor] gave me blood pressure medication, which brought it right back down to normal."

CHRIS

If you do take this medication, you have to be checked by your physician regularly. Doctors sometimes suggest you use cyclosporine for up to 2 years, but many experts feel that the best and safest way to use it is in short courses of up to 12 weeks at a time.

Methotrexate

Methotrexate has been used to treat psoriasis since the late 1960s. It works because it interferes with the body's ability to produce folate, a vitamin that encourages the growth of new skin cells. It also has a direct anti-inflammatory action on the skin by helping to control the overactive white blood cells associated with psoriasis. You take methotrexate once a week, usually in pill form.

You might respond to treatment within 2 or 3 weeks, but more likely it will take 8 to 12 weeks to notice a difference in your condition. There are no standard approaches to therapy. Some dermatologists prefer to start with a low "test dose" of one or two pills before increasing the amount of methotrexate you're taking.

! [**KEY POINT**]

Don't drink alcohol or take sulfa drugs while you're on methotrexate. You should also make every effort to avoid pregnancy. If you develop yellow skin and eyes (i.e., jaundice), develop a cough or start to bruise very easily, stop taking your methotrexate and consult your doctor.

Even though methotrexate has a long list of downsides (see below), it can provide effective relief from psoriasis skin symptoms for years—even decades. Other potential upsides of methotrexate are that it works for psoriatic arthritis and may decrease your risk of heart disease.

However, methotrexate doesn't work well for, or isn't tolerated by, about two-thirds of the people who take it. One of this drug's main side effects is liver damage. Another is stomach upset, which you can potentially avoid by taking a folate supplement. Although the supplement might reduce the effectiveness of methotrexate, it makes it more pleasant, allowing you to take this medication for a much longer period of time. If you're bothered by stomach upset with oral methotrexate, ask your doctor about scheduling regular methotrexate injections instead.

"[Methotrexate] made me feel like I had the flu. You're dragged out and nauseous. The only thing that I found to alleviate the nausea was you always had to have something in your stomach."

CHRIS

Your physician will probably not prescribe methotrexate for you, or give you a very low dose, if you have a low blood cell count, are obese, have liver disease, are diabetic, are an older adult or are struggling with alcoholism. Methotrexate should never be used by a woman who is pregnant, since it can harm a fetus, and any man who wants to father a child should not try until he's been off this drug for at least 1 month.

A Word from Dr. Papp

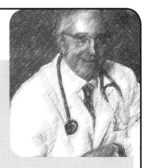

A Word About Risk

Although the risks involved in certain psoriasis treatments may worry you at first, keep in mind that you're no stranger to risk—you take risks every day.

Think about driving a car: you know there's always the risk of an accident, even though you reduce that risk by making sure that your car is in good mechanical shape, you're alert and obey the rules of the road. You also protect yourself by wearing a seat belt and buying a car with air bags. But, of course, none of this guarantees you won't be injured in an accident.

On the other hand, driving has many benefits. Cars get you places quickly and let you transport items that would be impossible to carry on a bicycle or by foot.

When you take a medication, it's much the same. There are risks, but there are also all sorts of safety measures in place to protect you. Health authorities are always monitoring information on drug safety. If the benefit of a medication turns out to be too small, or if the risk of harm is too great, it won't be approved or it will be withdrawn from the market.

No medication works for 100 percent of people, so there's a chance that you won't get better and that you'll develop some side effects. On the other hand, if the treatment helps you, the benefits can be huge. The decision you and your doctor face is always whether the benefits of a medication justify the risk of something bad happening.

Before you make any decisions, discuss all of your options with your doctor and ask questions about the benefits and risk of your possible treatments (see page 63). Remember that the treatment choice you ultimately make is very personal, so take the time to make sure you're comfortable with it—it's your body and health.

Biologics

Biologics are drugs made from living cells that are purified so they can be used as medicines. Although using biologic drugs to treat psoriasis is relatively new, biologics have been around for a while. Two examples of more familiar, older biologics are insulin and certain vaccines.

Like cyclosporine and methotrexate, biologics act on the immune system, but they are different in that they are targeted—they are specially designed to block one step in the damaging series of events that lead to psoriasis. Biologics also have to be taken by injection because their large, delicate molecules would be digested very quickly by your body if you ingested them in pill or capsule form.

There are five biologic drugs for psoriasis in Canada: adalimumab (Humira), etanercept (Enbrel), infliximab (Remicade), alefacept (Amevive) and ustekinumab (Stelara). Biologics are offering new hope to people with psoriasis by providing faster and better disease control than many other drugs on the market. However, as with all drugs for psoriasis, biologics also have some safety concerns, such as their ability to increase the risk of developing cancer, infections and other diseases that affect the immune system. For a quick reference to biologics, see page 109.

Before your doctor can give you a biologic, you'll have to answer some questions and undergo a few tests to see if you are eligible to take one of these drugs (see Who Shouldn't Take Biologics? on page 86). Your doctor will start by giving you a full physical exam and asking about your health and vaccination history. Then he or she will assess how severe your psoriasis is. Your liver and kidney function will be checked, and you may be tested for **hepatitis** B and C, the **human immunodeficiency virus (HIV)** and tuberculosis.

Your doctor may also test your blood sugar levels, give you a chest X-ray and look for signs of inflammation in your blood. If you and your doctor decide that biologics are a good option for you, your doctor will develop a plan to transition you from your current medication to whichever biologic drug will work best for you. Once you're on a biologic, your doctor will want to see you every few months to make sure you're responding well to your treatment and to check your blood.

You should contact your doctor between regular visits if you get sick with something worse than the common cold. If you do get very sick, it's important that you stop taking your biologic drug until your symptoms have subsided and the treatments for your illness are done (e.g., your fever is gone and your antibiotics are finished). If you continue to feel sick, see your dermatologist before restarting your treatment.

Who Shouldn't Take Biologics?
Because of their potential side effects, biologics aren't for everybody. For example, adalimumab, etanercept and infliximab haven't been studied much in women who are pregnant or breastfeeding, so you may be taken off these drugs if you tell your doctor that you're thinking of becoming pregnant. People with recurring infections, chronic ulcers, a history of cancer, heart failure, tuberculosis, multiple sclerosis or liver disease may also be at greater risk if they start on a biologic.

However, sometimes doctors prescribe biologics to people in these groups if the benefits of using them outweigh their risks. As always, you should work with your physician to come up with a treatment plan that suits your specific needs and goals.

Adalimumab, Etanercept and Infliximab: The Anti-TNF Drugs

Adalimumab, etanercept and infliximab block tumor necrosis factor (TNF), a protein in your body whose job is to promote inflammation (for more on inflammation, see the More Detail box on page 30). All these drugs can provide fast and effective relief, including clearing up your plaques completely, and they can be used to treat psoriatic arthritis. They are also used to control rheumatoid arthritis, ankylosing spondylitis and inflammatory bowel disease (Crohn's disease and ulcerative colitis), and have been used for nearly two decades by millions of people.

If you take adalimumab, you might start to see an improvement in your condition after 3 or 4 weeks of treatment, with a full benefit by week 16. About 70 to 75 percent of people respond well to this medication within these first 16 weeks, but the number tends to drop off a little after 6 months to a year of treatment.

You inject this drug under your skin every other week (see Help Yourself to Easier Injections on page 89), and it's best used regularly— if you take long breaks from your adalimumab, you increase the chances that it will stop working. You may experience welts and hives where you inject adalimumab or on other parts of your body. Antihistamines can sometimes reduce the severity of these reactions, which tend to persist or get worse with each injection.

Figure 7.3 How do psoriasis treatments help?

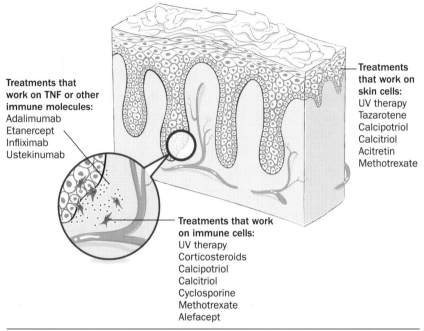

Treatments that work on TNF or other immune molecules:
Adalimumab
Etanercept
Infliximab
Ustekinumab

Treatments that work on skin cells:
UV therapy
Tazarotene
Calcipotriol
Calcitriol
Acitretin
Methotrexate

Treatments that work on immune cells:
UV therapy
Corticosteroids
Calcipotriol
Calcitriol
Cyclosporine
Methotrexate
Alefacept

Treatments for psoriasis work in several different ways. Some target the immune cells, while others act on skin cells or the faulty immune molecules. Some treatments, such as UV therapy, have more than one helpful effect.

Help Yourself to Easier Injections [SELF-HELP]

It's normal to be afraid of needles, especially ones that you have to give yourself—after all, one of your strongest natural instincts is to protect yourself from pain! But truthfully, putting a needle into your skin doesn't really hurt. The needle is so small and the process so fast that most people hardly feel anything. Here are some secrets to making self-injection as pain-free as possible:

1. Pinch the skin on your abdomen or thigh and push the needle in at a 45-degree angle. If you have a little more fat, you can put the needle straight in.
2. If the technique in Step 1 doesn't reduce the pain enough for you, you can apply an ice cube to the injection site for about 10 seconds to numb the skin before the needle goes in.
3. Make sure that the syringe and medication are at room temperature. Cold liquids cause more discomfort.
4. Inject the medication slowly to minimize the slight burning sensation that can accompany the shot.
5. If all else fails and you just can't bring yourself to inject your medication, there's nothing wrong with asking a family member, neighbor or friend to do it for you!

Etanercept was one of the first biologics approved for treating psoriasis and is probably one of the most flexible, allowing some people to see improvements in their psoriasis or psoriatic arthritis on very low doses or with intermittent use. Like adalimumab, etanercept is injected under the skin. It can take a bit longer to work than adalimumab and infliximab. You don't usually see significant improvements in your symptoms until you've been on it for 4 to 6 weeks, and it may take about 6 months to experience etanercept's full benefit.

About 55 to 65 percent of people do really well on etanercept in the first 3 months, but some people find that etanercept loses its effectiveness after 1 or 2 years. You inject etanercept under your skin once or twice a week. You can have injection-site reactions, such as red marks or hives. However, these reactions are very uncommon and when they do occur they often go away without any treatment.

Infliximab is not an injection. It needs to be infused into a vein at a specialized infusion clinic. It usually works very quickly and very well for both psoriasis and psoriatic arthritis. You'll start with three infusions in a row: one right away, the second 2 weeks later and the third on week 6 of your treatment. After that, you'll get an infusion every 8 weeks, although many people need treatment every 6 weeks to maintain good control of their psoriasis. About 80 percent of patients respond well to infliximab within the first 10 weeks of treatment, but some people stop responding well after 1 or 2 years of therapy, or after taking long breaks from it.

You can take comfort in knowing that you will never be asked to infuse yourself. Infusion clinics are staffed by experienced healthcare professionals who are specially trained in this type of procedure. When you go for your infusion, a needle will be placed into a vein in your arm. The needle is attached to a sterilized plastic hose that is connected to a pump or bag containing your medication. The speed at which your medication is infused is controlled by a valve or the intravenous pump. It usually takes 2 to 4 hours to complete an infusion.

Fortunately, reactions to infused medications are uncommon, and the infusion clinic staff have drugs on hand that can reverse bad reactions. These reactions can include widespread welts and hives, severe chest pains or headaches, and more severe allergic reactions.

However, most of the time, reactions can be stopped simply by slowing down the infusion or discontinuing it for a few minutes. The majority of infusion reactions are mild and include itching, headache, muscle aches or chills.

All of the anti-TNF drugs (adalimumab, etanercept and infliximab) work in similar ways, and they all seem to have the potential for causing certain very rare side effects. These side effects can be serious if they do occur, and include tuberculosis and other infectious diseases, heart problems and certain kinds of cancer. The anti-TNF drugs can also, strangely, cause psoriasis to flare, even in people who are taking them for other reasons and who never experienced psoriasis before!

If you develop large lymph nodes (what most people call "swollen glands"), bumps or open sores that don't heal, a severe rash or hives, burning during urination, sore gums or teeth, a persistent cough, a fever, wounds with redness around the edges, persistent tingling sensations, numbness, double or blurred vision, or weakness in your arms or legs on an anti-TNF drug, contact your doctor immediately. You should also call your physician if you gain weight rapidly, become very pale or start to bruise easily.

Because these side effects happen so infrequently, it's hard to say which of these drugs has the best safety record overall. But it's worth keeping in mind that none of the biologics cause frequent side effects, such as the liver or kidney damage that are common in people taking some of the oral systemic medications described on pages 79 to 83.

Nail Psoriasis—Can Biologics Help? [MORE DETAIL]

Nail psoriasis has always been tricky to treat. In the past, doctors have tried injecting medication under the nail, which is painful, or prescribing topical creams, which don't work well because they can't penetrate the nail. More recently, the medical community has started to use biologic drugs to treat severe nail psoriasis, with some success. So far, adalimumab, etanercept and infliximab seem to provide the most effective relief.

Alefacept

Alefacept is the only biologic drug in Canada that acts directly on white blood cells. It was the first biologic to be approved for treating more severe psoriasis. It appears to be quite safe for most people, but it's not as effective as the anti-TNF drugs. Alefacept is either self-injected or injected by a nurse into the muscle once a week for 12 weeks.

Low lymphocyte (a type of white blood cell) counts are common side effects of alefacept, so you need to have your blood checked every 2 weeks to make sure that your lymphocyte count isn't too low. If you develop a fever or need antibiotics to treat an infection, you should stop taking alefacept until your fever is gone or you've finished your antibiotics and are feeling better.

Unlike other biologics, alefacept is supposed to be used for only short periods of time, much like phototherapy, which is used until your symptoms clear up and then stopped. Alefacept has also been shown to be more effective when combined with UVB therapy (see Combination Therapies on page 95). Alefacept works in about 10 to 20 percent of people and can take up to 14 weeks to provide its full benefit. Those who do very well on alefacept have treatments every 3 to 12 months and show consistent improvement, but the biggest challenge with this drug is that we can't yet predict who will respond well to it.

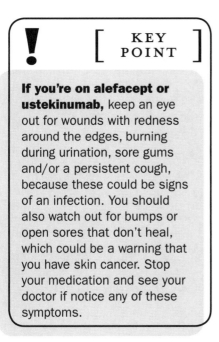

[KEY POINT]

If you're on alefacept or ustekinumab, keep an eye out for wounds with redness around the edges, burning during urination, sore gums and/or a persistent cough, because these could be signs of an infection. You should also watch out for bumps or open sores that don't heal, which could be a warning that you have skin cancer. Stop your medication and see your doctor if notice any of these symptoms.

Ustekinumab

Ustekinumab is very effective in treating moderate to severe psoriasis. This relatively new biologic drug targets specific proteins involved in regulating your immune response. These proteins are called interleukin-12 and interleukin-23. Researchers think that most of ustekinumab's effectiveness is based on its ability to block interleukin-23.

There is some concern that, as with all treatments for psoriasis, there might be a slightly increased risk of infections with ustekinumab. At this point, we don't know all the facts and can't say with any certainty whether or not this drug has a big impact on risk of infection. There is also some concern with a medication related to ustekinumab, but not yet on the market, that there is an increased risk of heart attacks or strokes. Until we know more about these medications, it may be advisable to avoid treatment with anti-interleukin-12 and anti-interleukin-23 medications if your risk of heart attack or stroke is high (e.g., you have uncontrolled high blood pressure, cholesterol or diabetes, or have had a recent stroke or heart attack).

Ustekinumab is injected under your skin once every 8 to 12 weeks. Many doctors prefer to give you the injections, so they can track your response to the drug and your overall health status. A single injection of ustekinumab gives many people complete clearance after anywhere from 2 to 6 weeks, with benefits lasting many months. However, some people take 12 to 16 weeks to respond, and some don't respond at all.

Because ustekinumab is the newest of the biologics and it's not used for diseases other than psoriasis, much less is known about its long-term safety, compared with other treatments. Injection-site reactions occur infrequently and tend to be local redness or itching. It is not known how effective ustekinumab is in treating psoriatic arthritis, but there are studies underway to test this and to learn more about peoples' experience with this new biologic drug.

Drugs for Psoriatic Arthritis [**MORE DETAIL**]

Six drugs are currently used in Canada for psoriatic arthritis:
- Cyclosporine
- Methotrexate
- Adalimumab
- Etanercept
- Infliximab
- Golimumab (another biologic related to adalimumab, etanercept and infliximab)

Combination Therapies—Strength in Numbers

Sometimes when two treatments are used as **combination therapy**, they work better than they would alone. For example, combining two topical treatments is usually even more effective than using just one. Plus, it can result in fewer side effects because you're not exposing your skin to the same medication over and over again.

A common topical combination that tends to work well—especially for controlling mild plaque psoriasis—is a mixture of calcipotriol with betamethasone (a topical steroid). However, this steroid–vitamin D combination, called Dovobet, can't be used in facial, flexural and genital psoriasis.

Steroids and tazarotene (a topical retinoid) are also sometimes combined, as are steroids and water-in-oil cream, or salicylic acid. Salicylic acid is a drug that removes psoriasis scaling so that other medications can more easily reach underneath thick layers of skin. It is often added to shampoos, lotions, creams and ointments. It shouldn't be applied in high concentrations over large areas of your body, as it can cause ringing in your ears or high blood acidity (metabolic acidosis). This drug also shouldn't be used in babies or young children. It's rare to develop an allergy to salicylic acid, but this medication can cause an asthma-like reaction in some people.

If you have more severe psoriasis, your physician may choose to combine non-topical treatments with other therapies. Methotrexate is often used in combination with light therapy, and acitretin (an oral retinoid) can be combined with light therapy, vitamin D–based medication or biologics to achieve better results. However, because acitretin can harm a fetus, women may be prescribed a combination of light therapy plus vitamin D-based medication or tazarotene.

Help Yourself to Better Drug Safety

[SELF-HELP]

- Always carry a list of your medications with you.
- If you're having a problem with your psoriasis medication, stop taking it and call your physician immediately.
- Never take a non-prescription medication, herb or supplement without first checking to see whether it interacts with your psoriasis medication.
- If you miss a dose of your medication, don't double up on the next dose.
- Always tell your doctors and pharmacists about any other medications, herbs or supplements you are on.
- Stay organized at home and on-the-go to avoid missing doses or mixing up medications—try using a pill organizer, and keep as many of your medications in once place as possible (e.g., store medications that don't need to be refrigerated together on their own shelf, and store medications that need to be refrigerated in a separate container, such as a clearly labeled box).
- Be sure to re-order your medication before it runs out.

Is Your Treatment Working? Knowing When to Ask for a Change

The medical community figures out whether a drug works or not by conducting clinical trials (see page 98). Clinical trials are studies designed in very specific ways to carefully test new therapies. The reason this is important is that psoriasis—even very bad psoriasis—can sometimes get better on its own, which is why many alternative therapies seem to "cure" this and other conditions.

> "I was part of an immigrant family that didn't have these wonderful medical plans, so all the medication that was ever purchased was through the hard work of my parents or myself."
>
> ANONYMOUS PATIENT

However, just because a drug works in a clinical trial doesn't mean that it will work for your skin. In real-life, success is not about the numbers—it's about you. Are you happy with the results of your treatment? Regardless of what your doctor or study results say, if you don't feel that your treatment is working well enough, ask to explore other options. There are now so many psoriasis therapies available that if one isn't doing the trick, it's worth trying another.

Funding Your Treatment: Plenty of Options

One of the biggest challenges that people with psoriasis face is the cost of their treatment. For example, the bill for a biologic typically comes in at $20,000 a year—and sometimes as much as $50,000. Fortunately, there are some potential ways to get funding for your treatment if you can't afford to pay for it yourself.

Government Funding

As we mentioned in Chapter 5 (see page 50), certain groups of people qualify for government drug benefits, plus other funding programs specific to your province or territory may be available to you. We recommend that you explore the information listed under Canada's Healthcare System and Health Benefits in the Resources section of this book (see page 213) to find out if you qualify for federal, provincial or territorial financial assistance.

Clinical Trials

Another way you might be able to fund your treatment is by joining a clinical trial, which is a health-related study to test new therapies on people. To be considered for a clinical trial, you have to meet certain criteria, such as being a certain age or gender, or having certain symptoms.

If you are accepted into a trial, you'll have to sign an informed consent sheet that explains all the benefits and risks of participating in the study. It's important to read the informed consent sheet and make sure you understand everything it says before signing it.

Then, in many cases, you'll be randomly assigned to one of two groups—the treatment group or the placebo group. The treatment group receives the new medication that's being tested, while the placebo group—also called the control group—is given a substance that may look like the drug being tested but has no medicinal properties. This means that you stand a chance of being assigned to the placebo group and will remain untreated for the duration of the clinical trial (see More Detail box on page 100).

Scientists do this to see if the medication that they're testing is actually helping patients. If the people in the treatment group are no better off than the people in the placebo group by the end of the study, researchers will know that the drug didn't actually do its job and that taking it is similar to receiving no treatment at all.

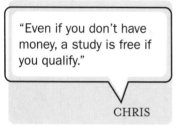

"Even if you don't have money, a study is free if you qualify."

CHRIS

However, there are two things to keep in mind, even if you are given the placebo. First, you can always leave the trial and go back to another treatment. Second, many trials have a second stage, where there is no placebo group and everyone in the study gets the drug being tested. People in this kind of trial still get the study drug for free, sometimes for many months or years.

Studies also sometimes compare two drugs, so you may be put into a treatment group that is receiving an older medication that has already been on the market for a while.

You can find out about clinical trials that are currently running through clinicaltrials.gov or researchtrials.org, but to sign up for one, you need to get connected with a doctor who is involved in these kinds of studies. If your family physician or dermatologist doesn't conduct this type of research, you can ask for a referral to someone who does.

The Benefits and Risks of Clinical Trials

[**MORE DETAIL**]

Joining a clinical trial to get free treatment might seem like a perfect solution, but risks come along with the many benefits of participating in this kind of study. Keep in mind that clinical trials are also the only way new therapies can be developed. Even if the drug you're trying doesn't work for you, it could work for someone else.

Clinical Trial Benefits	Clinical Trial Risks
Your treatment is free	You could end up in the placebo group (i.e., you might not receive the drug that's being tested)
You gain access to the latest treatments	If you're in the treatment group, you could experience side effects from the medication you are put on, or you may find the drug does not work for you
You are usually treated at the best facilities and receive expert care	A large time commitment might be involved, including trips to where the study is being conducted, hospital stays, multiple treatments and complex dosage requirements
You will be helping others by contributing to medical research	Even if the drug works for you, you might end up having to go off it once the trial is finished

Private Insurance

A very common option is to get funding for treatment through a private insurance plan. If you don't have a plan, you can purchase one, or you might already be covered under your spouse's work policy. Be aware, though, that many insurance companies won't cover treatments for pre-existing conditions (i.e., conditions that you had before you purchased the plan).

However, every insurer is different, so it's best to call around and compare which companies offer you the best deal. Once you're insured, you may also need a note from your doctor to access funding for more expensive or newer drugs, such as biologics.

Drug Company Assistance

Some drug companies are working on ways to help foot the bill for some of their most expensive treatments and have begun patient support programs that help with drug costs, as well as provide education and advice. Bear in mind that these programs are purely voluntary for each company, and their policies can change at the company's discretion. Patient support programs also shouldn't be confused with the drug support that's available to qualifying people through their province, territory or private insurance. One way to find out about patient support programs is to ask your dermatologist about them, or read up on some of the current plans below.

Drug	Patient Support Program	Contact Information
Adalimumab (Humira)	Progress Program: Once you have your prescription for adalimumab, call to speak with a reimbursement specialist who can help you explore payment options	1-866-848-6472 1-866-8HUMIRA www.humira-progress.ca
Etanercept (Enbrel)	Enliven Support Services: Once you have a prescription for etanercept, contact the program for more details; you can ask your doctor to enrol you or you can enrol yourself online—assistance is based on a financial means-based evaluation and is reassessed each year	1-877-936-2735 1-877-9ENBREL www.enbrel.ca
Infliximab (Remicade)	Bioadvance Program: Once you have a prescription for infliximab, you can access financial aid to help find reimbursement options for your medication as well as help with insurance claims	1-866-872-5774 https://bioadvance.ca
Golimumab (Simponi)	Bioadvance Program: Once you have a prescription for golimumab, you can access financial aid to help find reimbursement options for your medication as well as help with insurance claims	1-866-872-5774 https://bioadvance.ca
Ustekinumab (Stelara)	Johnson and Johnson Patient Assistance Foundation: Once you have a prescription for ustekinumab, you can apply online or you can request a mail-in application over the phone—assistance is based on your household size and annual gross income, and is given for up to 1 year at a time; after 1 year, you may reapply so that your situation can be reassessed	1-800-652-6227 www.jjpaf.org

Continued...

(cont.)

Drug	Patient Support Program	Contact Information
Alefacept (Amevive)	Once you have a prescription for alefacept, you can submit your insurance and financial information to the program—eligibility for and amount of support is determined on a case-by-case basis, and reimbursement is provided for a maximum of 3 to 4 weeks (i.e., the course of the treatment)	1-877-AMEVIVE 1-877-263-8483
Tacrolimus (Protopic)	Once you have a prescription for tacrolimus, you may be eligible for reimbursement, the amount of which is determined on a case-by-case basis	Speak with your physician to gain access to the program

Quick Reference Therapy Guide

Treatment	Pros	Cons	Who Shouldn't Use
Topical Treatments			
Topical steroids	Effective at relieving symptoms Helpful for people with mild psoriasis	Can cause skin-related side effects with frequent use May become less effective with frequent use May not help people with more severe psoriasis	Anyone who develops an allergy to steroids
Vitamin D ointments	Can be effective at relieving symptoms Helpful for people with moderate and severe psoriasis who aren't helped by steroids Won't cause long-term, irreversible skin damage Can reduce amount of steroids needed to achieve relief Calcitriol (not calcipotriol can be used continuously for one year Can be used in children	Generally not as effective as the most powerful steroids Can cause skin irritation, although calcitriol may be less irritating than calcipotriol Calcipotriol can cause high blood calcium levels in rare cases Not recommended for genital psoriasis Calcipotriol is not recommended for the face or skin folds (note: calcitriol is usually okay in these areas)	Anyone whose skin becomes too irritated

Continued...

Treatment	Pros	Cons	Who Shouldn't Use
Tacrolimus and pimecrolimus	Can be used on the face or skin folds where the skin is thin	Don't work well on areas of the body where the skin is thick	
Tazarotene	Effective at relieving symptoms Helpful for people with mild psoriasis	Can cause significant skin irritation Less helpful for people with more severe psoriasis	Anyone whose skin becomes too irritated
Moisturizers	Non-medicated way to control skin flaking, cracking, itching and bleeding Can reduce the amount of steroids needed to achieve relief Can control psoriasis completely if the condition is extremely mild and limited	Can cause allergic reactions, folliculitis, irritation or itching	Anyone who develops an allergy to moisturizers
Tar	Can help control psoriasis	Stains clothes Smells bad Could possibly increase the risk of developing cancer Can irritate skin	Anyone whose skin becomes too irritated Anyone who is allergic to tar

Continued...

Treatment	Pros	Cons	Who Shouldn't Use
Phototherapy			
Phototherapy	Can lead to the full relief of symptoms	Over-exposure can cause sunburn-like effects if not done properly	Anyone who has already had 200 PUVA sessions or skin cancer
		PUVA increases the risk of developing cancer, and the long-term safety of UVB has not been determined	Anyone with lupus, photodermatosis or a history of cancer
		PUVA can lead to skin aging and freckling	Anyone whose psoriasis gets worse on phototherapy
		Inconvenient and not always accessible	
Systemic Treatments			
Acitretin	Effective	Can harm a fetus up to 3 years after you stop taking it	Women who are pregnant or thinking of becoming pregnant within 3 years
	Helps phototherapy work better and reduces the amount of necessary UV ray exposure	Can cause chapped, dry lips, dry skin and dry eyes	Women in their child-bearing years who have trouble using birth control reliably
		Can raise triglyceride levels	
		Can cause bone abnormalities	
		Best used in combination with other treatments	
		Can cause stiff joints and sore muscles	
		Can cause hair loss	
		Can't drink alcohol or take vitamin A supplements while on acetretin	

Continued...

Treatment	Pros	Cons	Who Shouldn't Use
Cyclosporine	Can effectively control symptoms Can be used continuously for up to 2 years	Can cause irreversible kidney damage Can cause high blood pressure and elevated triglycerides Can increase the risk of developing skin cancer and lymphoma Requires you to have your kidney function, blood pressure and triglycerides checked regularly Can cause temporary tingling in the fingers, toes, lips and face Can cause headaches, muscle aches or stomach upset	Anyone who is bothered by cyclosporine's side effects

Continued...

Treatment	Pros	Cons	Who Shouldn't Use
Methotrexate	Can be effective at controlling symptoms Can potentially be used consistently for decades	Doesn't work as well as cyclosporine over a 12-week period Can cause liver damage Requires you to have occasional liver biopsies Can cause a reduction in the number of red and white blood cells and platelets Can cause lung damage Slightly increases the risk of developing lymphoma and low blood cell counts Can cause significant nausea Can harm a fetus or cause miscarriage Can cause a condition that weakens and thins bones	Women who are pregnant Men who want to conceive with their partner within 1 month of being on methotrexate Anyone with a low blood cell count Anyone who is obese Anyone who has liver disease Anyone who is diabetic Anyone consuming alcohol

Continued...

Treatment	Pros	Cons	Who Shouldn't Use
Adalimumab	Can provide fast and effective relief from symptoms Can treat psoriatic arthritis and inflammatory bowel disease Can treat nail psoriasis	Can stop working if you stop using it for a long time Can cause injection reactions Can lose its effectiveness after 1 or 2 years	Women who are pregnant or thinking of becoming pregnant Anyone with recurring infections Anyone with chronic ulcers Anyone with a history of cancer, or, specifically, lymphoma Anyone with heart failure Anyone with tuberculosis Anyone with multiple sclerosis Anyone with liver disease

Continued...

Treatment	Pros	Cons	Who Shouldn't Use
Alefacept	Can provide fast and effective relief from symptoms The only biologic that allows patients to go off treatment once their psoriasis is cleared to their satisfaction	Not as effective as the other biologics Sometimes combined with UVB therapy Can cause infections Can cause low lymphocyte counts You need to have your blood checked every 2 weeks during treatment	Anyone with a fever or who is on antibiotics Anyone who has had cancer, or, specifically, lymphoma

Continued...

Treatment	Pros	Cons	Who Shouldn't Use
Etanercept	Can provide fast and effective relief from symptoms Can treat psoriatic arthritis and inflammatory bowel disease Can treat nail psoriasis	Can take longer to work than adalimumab and infliximab Can cause injection reactions Can slowly lose its effectiveness after 1 or 2 years	Women who are pregnant or thinking of becoming pregnant Anyone with recurring infections Anyone with chronic ulcers Anyone with a history of cancer, or, specifically, lymphoma Anyone with heart failure Anyone with tuberculosis Anyone with multiple sclerosis Anyone with liver disease

Continued...

Treatment	Pros	Cons	Who Shouldn't Use
Infliximab	Can provide fast and effective relief from symptoms Has been around longer than adalimumab and used more extensively in treating flares Can treat psoriatic arthritis and inflammatory bowel disease Can treat nail psoriasis	Can lose its effectiveness after 1 or 2 years or after long breaks from using it Has to be infused Can cause infusion reactions	Women who are pregnant or thinking of becoming pregnant Anyone with recurring infections Anyone with chronic ulcers Anyone with a history of cancer, or, specifically, lymphoma Anyone with heart failure Anyone with tuberculosis Anyone with multiple sclerosis Anyone with liver disease
Ustekinumab	Effective for skin psoriasis	Not a lot of information on ustekinumab's long-term safety	Anyone with cancer Anyone with an infection Anyone who has had lymphoma

Chapter 8

how you can help yourself

What Happens in This Chapter
- Reducing your pain and itch
- Overcoming emotional and financial challenges
- Maintaining your overall health
- How to make treatment time easier

Although your psoriasis might make you feel helpless sometimes, there are actually lots of things you can do to ease your worry and physical discomfort. By following a few tips and tricks, you can reduce your stress, medication costs, and itch and pain, and make treatment time easier.

Reducing Physical Discomfort

Although taking your medication is always the first and most important step in keeping your pain and itch under control, there are a few other things you can do to ease your physical discomfort.

Reducing the Itch

If your psoriasis is itchy, there are ways to minimize or stop that nagging irritation. Scratching only makes itching worse, so here are some better ways to find relief:

- If you find that you scratch in your sleep, ask your physician if you can take antihistamines, such as diphenhydramine (Benadryl) or hydroxyzine (Atarax), before going to bed.
- Some people find that lotions soothe the itch a bit, as well as soften the skin so that it is less likely to split and bleed.
- Stay cool—heat makes the itch worse.
- Cover your skin to make sure it doesn't dry out and become more irritated.
- If you have a few pustules, draining them with a sterilized pin can reduce their itch or pain.
- If you have just one area that is a problem, putting on an ice cube for a few seconds will almost instantly remove the itch.

"Be strong—don't scratch! You just get used to not scratching. It feels sometimes like little pins and needles, but once you've taught yourself not to scratch, you carry on. If you put some kind of lotion or something on, it takes care of it."

TOM

Preventing and Treating Cracks and Fissures

Because psoriasis thickens your skin, it's more likely to crack. Keeping your skin very moisturized will go a long way toward making it softer and more supple, and will help prevent it from developing painful fissures. If you do develop a fissure, apply a thick moisturizer, such as Vaseline, Bag Balm, udder cream or lanolin, and cover the area with a light cotton sock or glove—leaving the moisturizer on overnight works even better! You can also apply a simple tape dressing over your fissure to reduce the pain and increase healing.

Avoiding Flare Triggers

One of the best ways to keep your physical discomfort to a minimum is to reduce your chances of flaring. Each person with psoriasis has different flare triggers. They can include hormonal changes, skin injury, weather, certain medications or a combination of stressful life circustances. You can become familiar with your triggers and create a plan to avoid them where possible by tracking them in the symptom diary on page 228. Read pages 202 to 203 for more information on how to prevent flares.

Overcoming Emotional Challenges

Although it may seem impossible at times, you truly can overcome the social and emotional challenges of your psoriasis and have a happy and productive life, just like many other people have before you. Chapter 5 gave you tips on how to prepare for your psoriasis journey. If you're feeling down, try turning to Chapter 11 for some ideas on how to handle the stress you're dealing with. Read Chapter 13 for information on how to help a child with psoriasis cope with his or her feelings.

"There's so much to think about. When you're really bad, you have to stand on paper so you can get dressed and all of your scales can fall off. Everything is a chore, but you do get used to it."

MARGIE

Overcoming Financial Challenges

There are so many effective psoriasis treatments now, but some of them can be quite expensive—especially biologic drugs, which can be the only way to relieve many cases of more severe psoriasis. Although financial assistance isn't always an option, there are a few ways to get funding for costlier psoriasis medications. Read page 98 to learn about drug financing options.

Maintaining Good Overall Health

It's much easier to weather the ups and downs of psoriasis if your overall health is good. Eating nutritious food, exercising, socializing and getting enough sleep can all help you feel better not only physically, but also mentally. Even though lifestyle changes are hard to make, they're always worth it. For more information on how to improve your well-being, read pages 128 to 137.

Making Treatment Time Easier

It's common to have questions about how to use your medication once you get it home—instructions that seem straightforward in your doctor's office are often less clear when you're faced with the reality of applying a cream, swallowing a pill or giving yourself an injection.

Fortunately, no matter what your psoriasis therapy regimen is, there are ways to make treatments easier. Read pages 66 to 69 to find out the secrets to simpler topical application, and for advice on how to give yourself an injection, read page 89. For information on how to make treatments less stressful for kids, read Chapter 13, and for drug safety tips, read the Self-Help box on page 96.

Chapter 9

complementary approaches to managing psoriasis

What Happens in This Chapter
- Which complementary psoriasis treatments do and don't work
- The importance of lifestyle changes

While some complementary psoriasis treatments don't work, others show potential. Psychological therapy, balneotherapy (a combination of salt water and UV light), and certain herbs and vitamins are a few approaches to managing psoriasis that have some scientific backup and may be worth a try. However, if a complementary approach isn't working, the same rules apply as for conventional treatments: don't suffer in silence. See your physician and keep working to find a medicine that will help you. It's also important to improve your overall health as much as possible by exercising, eating healthy food, getting enough sleep and quitting smoking and drinking.

Introduction

At some point you might become curious about complementary approaches to managing your psoriasis. Complementary therapies are, generally speaking, not as widely researched or as well funded as conventional treatments, and the studies that do exist are often not up to the standard of conventional drug trials. This means that we don't always know about side effects, interactions with conventional drugs or how people with different diseases might react to complementary treatments, so be cautious. A therapy isn't safe just because it's "natural" (the natural world contains some of our most powerful poisons).

There are, however, quite a few studies on complementary treatments, and the body of evidence giving clear hints about which do and don't work is steadily growing. In this chapter, we tell you which remedies may have some potential and which ones probably won't help you.

You may be surprised that we're willing to give space to therapies that don't work—or where the scientific evidence is a bit thin. Our thinking is that anyone with a chronic, important illness such as psoriasis will be inundated by advice from friends, alternative health practitioners and the Internet. To make good decisions you need to know the truth about the most common "psoriasis cures" that you'll hear about. If they're going to waste your money, raise false hopes and delay you getting access to something that might help you, we want you to know the facts.

Complementary Treatments With Some Scientific Backup

In this section you'll learn about complementary psoriasis approaches that have shown some potential in scientific studies. Although these treatments need to be studied further before they can be recommended regularly to patients, you may find one of them works for you.

Psychological Therapies

There is a lot of scientific evidence showing that psychological therapies can have a big impact on your psoriasis experience. Study after study has found that interventions such as **meditation**, relaxation techniques, support groups and counseling may not only help you feel better emotionally, but also physically.

A British study published in the *British Journal of Dermatology* in 2002 illustrates this phenomenon beautifully. Researchers provided people receiving phototherapy for their psoriasis with six sessions of group cognitive-behavioural therapy. The sessions included education about their disease, instruction on stress reduction techniques, and ways to deal with low self-esteem and the reactions of others to their condition. At the end of 6 weeks, the people in group therapy were far less depressed and anxious than a group of similar people who didn't receive counseling, which is perhaps to be expected. However, what was interesting was that the phototherapy actually worked better in the people who had received counseling: the skin of these people skin cleared faster and remained clear longer. Even 6 months later, the people who had received counseling in addition to phototherapy were doing better than those who only received phototherapy.

Similar results were seen in another British study published a year later in the *Archives of Dermatology,* which showed excessive worrying can affect how long it takes light therapy to work. The physicians running the study compared the length of time it took "high-level" or "low-level" worriers to achieve clearance of their psoriasis plaques. Remarkably, the skin of the people who worried a lot took almost twice as long to improve as the skin of people who worried less.

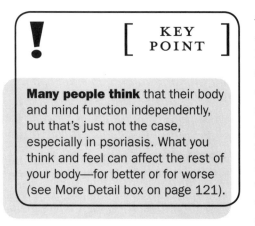

! [KEY POINT]

Many people think that their body and mind function independently, but that's just not the case, especially in psoriasis. What you think and feel can affect the rest of your body—for better or for worse (see More Detail box on page 121).

A study published in *Psychosomatic Medicine* in 1998 looked at the effects of mindfulness meditation on psoriasis. American researchers treated people with moderate to severe psoriasis with light therapy three times a week for approximately 13 weeks. Each time some of the participants went for UVB or PUVA treatments, they were asked to listen to an audiotape that guided them through a mindfulness-based stress reduction technique. The people who meditated responded more quickly to the treatment sessions and achieved clearance of their symptoms in less time than the people in a control group who didn't meditate.

If nothing else, these studies and others like them show why it's important to acknowledge and deal with your emotions when you're trying to heal. Of course, it can be tough to face your worries head-on, but there are so many benefits to lowering your stress levels. It makes sense to explore the options for managing your stress. If and when you feel ready, choose one that seems right for you. Read Chapter 11 to get some practical tips on how to work through your feelings and make your heart a little lighter (and, maybe, your skin a little clearer).

Stress: The Fight or Flight Response With Nowhere to Go [MORE DETAIL]

When we face a threat of some kind, a whole series of physical switches are flipped almost instantaneously—a reaction you've probably heard of called "the fight or flight response." Way back in history this reaction was designed to save us from physical danger—if a lion or neighboring tribe attacked, our bodies would kick into action and give us the power to fight back or run away. Here's what happens during the fight or flight response:

1. A part of the brain called the hypothalamus sounds an alarm and triggers your sympathetic nervous system.

2. Your sympathetic nervous system releases a hormone called adrenaline, which makes your heart beat faster, raises your blood pressure, slows your digestion and directs blood to your muscles so you have more power to defend yourself physically.

3. Your liver then releases stored sugar into your bloodstream to give you energy.

Running from the lion or the aggressive neighbors made use of the extra sugar, the pumping heart and the oxygenated muscles. When the danger was over, everything returned to normal. The problem with modern life is that our fight or flight response is constantly being triggered by all sorts of modern-day inconveniences, such as traffic, a tight work deadline or writing a test at school. We don't (usually) run or fight back so there's no way for our bodies to reset. Instead, we turn on the TV or reach for a drink. In effect, stress is a fight or flight response with nowhere to go. Over time, this constant assault on the body can affect a person's physical health.

Fish Oil

Fish oil has been researched quite a bit in the world of complementary medicine for treating all sorts of conditions—not just psoriasis. The reason there is a great deal of interest in the oils of cold-water fish, such as mackerel, sardine, salmon, kipper and herring, is that they have high amounts of omega-3, a type of "good" fat that may help reduce inflammation in the body.

However, so far, the research has been poorly designed and hasn't provided a lot of solid evidence to support using fish oil in psoriasis. There's also no clear information about how much might be needed to control psoriasis, although it seems that you may need large amounts of fish oil to feel its effects.

The few studies that have been done show that daily doses under 10 g taken for less than a month tend not to help people with psoriasis feel any better. Studies testing higher capsule doses or intravenous oil infusions for longer periods of time have been more positive, but it's still hard to be sure whether these treatments showed any true benefit. More research is needed before we'll know whether it's worth recommending fish oil to people with psoriasis, and what amounts may be effective. But here's what we do know:

- A British study published in 1988 in *The Lancet* showed that people with plaque psoriasis experienced significantly less itching, redness and scaling after 12 weeks on 18 g of fish oil per day than people who were taking a placebo of olive oil. However, the study had only 28 participants, so it's hard to draw conclusions.
- A European study published in 1993 followed people who had been hospitalized with severe guttate psoriasis and given 23.1 g of fish oil daily. These patients experienced a significantly greater improvement within 10 days than a group who received intravenous infusions containing omega-3 fats. However, the number of people who participated was quite small.
- A U.S. study published in 1990 in a journal called *Pharmacology & Therapeutics* reported that people with plaque psoriasis who received 9 g of fish oil daily for 3 weeks did not experience an improvement in their symptoms when compared to people who received olive oil supplements.

- A British study published in *The New England Journal of Medicine* in 1993 found that when study participants who had psoriasis took 1 g of fish oil daily for 4 months, they did not experience a significant decrease in their PASI scores when compared to people who received corn oil.

If you are allergic to fish, there are also **vegetarian** sources of omega-3 fats (see Chapter 10), such as flax oil supplements. However, you will need a lot more flax to get the same effect as with fish oil, because fish oil is easier for your body to process. If you want to try adding omega-3 supplements to your diet, it's best to work with a naturopathic or medical doctor who's familiar with prescribing them. Or see a dietitian or nutritionist who works regularly with people who have inflammatory conditions.

A Word from Dr. Papp

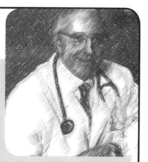

A Word About The Scientific Method

To minimize the chances that the results of a study are misleading, researchers aim to remove as much bias as possible from their methods. Bias is when we see patterns of events and think that they are related to or cause one another. Say, for example, that your psoriasis improved after you ate French fries. You might think that eating the fries cured your psoriasis, but in truth, it might be that your psoriasis was going to get better anyway. Or maybe a medication you took 2 weeks earlier finally started to work.

To reduce this bias, scientists test new treatments on large numbers of people (dozens, hundreds or thousands, instead of one or two). They also sometimes ask people not to take other medications while they are part of the study, and they design the study as best they can so that the results will be clear and easy to interpret.

Continued...

A Word from Dr. Papp (cont.)

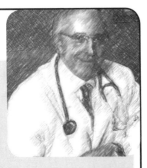

Scientists then divide their subjects into a treatment group, which gets the new therapy, and a control group, which gets a placebo—something that looks and feels like the treatment but doesn't have any medical effect. To further prevent bias, the study participants and researchers don't know which group is which. Who got the treatment and who got the placebo is only revealed at the end of the study, as the results are being analyzed.

When trying to understand whether treatments work or not another important concept is "significance." You may have noticed that medical researchers (and the descriptions of psoriasis research that we give in this book) talk about results being "significant." This word means something very different in the world of science than in everyday conversation. Significance in the scientific community is determined by a very strict set of rules and calculations to help researchers figure out whether or not the results of their studies are truly meaningful. This is particularly important when it comes to understanding whether complementary therapies do anything or not.

There are a couple of different kinds of significance—"statistical significance" and "clinical significance." If a result is "statistically significant," it is not likely to have occurred by chance. Because the results of any study can occur by random chance, researchers use statistics to figure out how likely it is that they have been fooled into believing that a certain treatment is helpful when it really isn't.

Continued...

A Word from Dr. Papp (cont.)

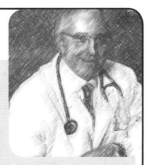

"Clinical significance" is the real-life effect of the drug on the patient—i.e., does it make the patient feel better or worse? Sometimes the results of a study are statistically significant (the drug is definitely clearing a patient's skin) but not clinically significant (the drug doesn't make the patient feel any better). Obviously, researchers hope that improvements seen with a drug will be statistically significant *and* clinically significant!

On the other hand, just because a treatment fails the statistical test for significance in a drug trial, it doesn't necessarily mean that the treatment is worthless—it could just mean that the effect is smaller or less consistent than the researchers expected when they started the study. Sometimes researchers have to go back and do a new study with many more subjects, just to be able to show whether there is a significant benefit.

These techniques—the scientific method—are used in pharmaceutical drug research. However, much of the research on non-pharmaceutical treatments don't use the scientific method. That's why it's hard to determine whether some of the alternative treatments for psoriasis are truly helpful.

Herbs and Psoriasis

Herbs can have a powerful effect on the body, so it's no surprise that researchers have looked at the potential of herbs for treating psoriasis. Two that have been studied are *Mahonia aquifolium* and neem.

Mahonia aquifolium (also called barberry or Oregon grape) is an evergreen shrub that contains berberine, a chemical with anti-inflammatory properties. Neem is a kind of evergreen tree found mostly in India. It has an active ingredient in its bark called nimbidin, which also happens to have powerful anti-inflammatory effects.

Both of these herbs were reported to reduce PASI scores in people with psoriasis. However, there is very little research backing up the claims, and the studies on *Mahonia aquifolium* and neem are poor in quality. Far more research is needed on these plants before they can be recommended to people with psoriasis.

Vitamin Supplements and Psoriasis

We know that vitamins can sometimes be helpful in treating certain conditions, but do they make any difference in psoriasis? The answer is, we're not sure yet. A few vitamins have been researched, such as topical vitamin B12 with avocado oil, oral vitamin D supplements and a combination of oral selenium, coenzyme Q10 and vitamin E. However, the studies are small and poorly designed, so it's not possible to tell for sure whether these vitamins are useful for treating psoriasis.

Balneotherapy

Balneotherapy is similar to light or phototherapy (see page 75), except that instead of combining psoralen with UVA or undergoing UVB treatments alone, you bathe in salt water before being exposed to UV rays. The idea behind this treatment is based on a traditional therapy that required people with psoriasis to vacation in sunny places with very salty water, such as the Dead Sea in Israel. The UV exposure that comes with sunbathing can certainly be helpful for psoriasis symptoms, but it's unclear whether the salt water also plays a role in healing skin.

One study published in 2007 followed the progress of people with psoriasis who soaked three times a week in very salty water for 20 minutes before being exposed to UVB. After 6 weeks of treatment, significantly more of these patients improved by 75 percent than a group of participants who received only UVB therapy.

Another study published in 2007 showed similar results, with a significant number of people on UVB and salt water therapy experiencing a 50 percent improvement in their symptoms. However, some studies show no improvement when salt water is added to light therapy, so more research is clearly needed before we know for sure whether balneotherapy is a valid treatment option.

> **!** **[KEY POINT]**
>
> **It's essential** to tell your medical and naturopathic doctors about all of the treatments that you're on, including light therapy, topical and systemic pharmaceutical drugs, herbs, vitamins, minerals and other supplements, such as fish oil. Just because a complementary treatment is "natural" doesn't mean that it can't be dangerous or interact with supplements, drugs and foods.

Complementary Treatments That Don't Work: Save Your Money

Many therapy claims you'll read about or hear about just aren't backed up by science. Here is a summary of treatments that are sometimes recommended with good intentions, but don't have any evidence to support them.

- **Zinc:** Because some people believe that zinc deficiency is linked to psoriasis, scientists have taken a look at whether zinc supplements can reverse the condition. The results were disappointing. For example, a study published in 1994 in *Cutis* showed that people with psoriasis showed no improvement when they supplemented their diet with zinc. Interestingly, there is a condition caused by zinc deficiency that can look like psoriasis in the groin and skin folds, but it's not related to psoriasis.
- **Selenium alone:** Although a combination of selenium, coenzyme Q10 and vitamin E supplements seems to help relieve symptoms in people with psoriasis (see page 126), taking selenium alone doesn't appear to have any healing effects. A study published in *Nutrition* in 2003 found no significant improvement in people with psoriasis who received this mineral.
- **Oleum horwathiensis:** These medicinal plants seemed to improve PASI scores in the treatment group of a small study published in the *Journal of International Medical Research* in 1991, but compared to placebo, the improvement wasn't significant.
- **Acupuncture and Chinese medicine:** These healing modalities have existed for centuries. There is no doubt that more and more research will be conducted to test their validity, but for now there is very little scientific backup to show that they are helpful to people with psoriasis.

Improving Your Overall Health: Live Well to Feel Well

Even if you aren't interested in trying complementary treatments to relieve your symptoms, making a few lifestyle changes can improve your overall health and may even help your psoriasis.

Exercise

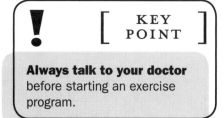

!   [KEY POINT]

Always talk to your doctor before starting an exercise program.

Why Exercise?

Exercising can be a challenge when you have psoriasis because heat and sweat can irritate your skin. Despite these obstacles, some of the patients who were kind enough to share their stories with us for this book have always exercised when they felt they were able to—one patient has loved swimming since childhood, and others play golf and bike. They enjoy the many benefits of working out regularly, including some that relate directly to their condition. Exercise can:

- Regulate your immunity when done in moderate (as opposed to extreme) amounts
- Make you feel happier and calmer
- Reduce your risk of developing heart disease
- Regulate your appetite
- Build your strength
- Help control your insulin levels
- Improve your sleep

Choosing Your Workout

The trick to exercising with psoriasis is to keep it simple and low impact. You don't have to be dripping with sweat to get fit and feel better! Try walking, or hiking along a shaded nature trail that doesn't have too many hills. Try a gentle stretch and strengthen class at your gym, ice-skating, rollerblading, low-intensity weight lifting, tai chi or **yoga**. In the case of yoga, be aware that there are many different kinds, some of which are more strenuous than others. Ask your local yoga center which type is right for you, and see the More Detail box on page 130.

What Is Yoga?

[**MORE DETAIL**]

Yoga originated in India and has been around since at least 3000 B.C. This ancient practice involves holding several physical postures to focus and calm the mind, as well as build strength, flexibility and balance. There are many different kinds of yoga, some of which may not be appropriate for you, depending on how severe your psoriasis is, how fit you are and how sensitive you are to heat.

The Hatha style is usually easier and a great place to start if you're new to yoga, but some studios can make their Hatha classes quite challenging. If you find sweating very uncomfortable or you aren't used to exercising regularly, it's best to try classes that are specifically labeled "gentle," "yin," "restorative" or, as in the Ahimsa method, "sukha." These types of lessons will help you become more familiar with your local yoga center and give you the chance to get to know instructors who deal regularly with beginners. Once you've attended a few low-intensity classes, feel free to discuss what other lessons might be right for you with a teacher you trust who has had a chance to observe you during your yoga practice.

Some studios also have programs designed specifically for beginners or people with health issues so they can build strength slowly and at their own pace.

Staying Comfortable During Exercise

If you worry that your skin will become irritated with exercise, there are ways to minimize your discomfort during and after a workout. It helps if you can stay well hydrated, avoid exercising in warm and humid environments and avoid over-exerting yourself. You can also reduce your chances of overheating by wearing loose-fitting cotton clothes.

If you find that certain movements during exercise cause your plaques to crack and bleed, you can apply moisturizer before your workout to improve your skin's flexibility. You may also want to modify some of the exercises during your workout. If you're taking a class, speak with your fitness instructor in advance and explain that you might not be able to do everything. Don't be shy about this—it's part of your exercise instructor's job to modify the training for students with various medical issues, so ask your teacher for suggestions on how to reduce the intensity of the movements that stretch your skin too much.

In addition, have a plan in case your skin becomes irritated or bleeds, so you're not caught off guard when you're exercising. Try packing a little first-aid kit in your gym bag with supplies such as bandages or a liquid bandage solution. Take a change of clothes, moisturizer and cab money in case you arrived by public transit but want to get home more quickly and privately. And remember—you can always take a break or stop your workout early if you find that you're in pain or too hot and uncomfortable.

If you have psoriatic arthritis, your joint pain might make exercising more challenging, although most people with this condition are able to tolerate regular workouts. The trick to exercising comfortably when you have joint pain is to start slowly and warm up. Avoid very heavy or extreme weight lifting because the strain on your tendons and ligaments might make your psoriatic arthritis worse.

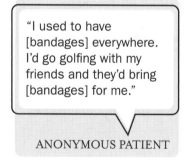

"I used to have [bandages] everywhere. I'd go golfing with my friends and they'd bring [bandages] for me."

ANONYMOUS PATIENT

Fitting Exercise Into Your Schedule

Even if you believe that exercise is important to your health, you're not alone if you feel it's hard to fit into your busy schedule, or you feel too out-of-shape to give it a try. Fortunately, there are ways to make exercise both achievable and fun. It also helps to be patient—building up strength takes a long time. Even if you don't feel the benefits of working out right away, stick with it and before you know it, you'll be healthier and have more energy. Below are some tips on how to stay physically active:

- Incorporate physical activity into your daily routine. Park farther away from a building's entrance so you get a bit of a walk. Climb the stairs instead of taking the elevator. Walk to the grocery store, or walk the dog.
- Carve out a slot of time each week to exercise. Join a class, sports league or group such as a hiking club, baseball team, yoga class or walking clinic.
- Do something you enjoy and encourage your family and friends to join in. Try kite flying, ice skating, playing physical games (e.g., catch, Frisbee, badminton), playing with a pet or taking a walk in your favorite neighborhood, mall, wooded area or park.

Get Enough Sleep

In the section on complementary treatments with potential (see page 119), we discussed why keeping your stress in check can help control your psoriasis. One way to minimize your stress level is to make sure you get enough sleep. Too little sleep starts a vicious cycle that causes the stress hormones in your body to increase, and those stress hormones, in turn, prevent you from sleeping properly.

Another great reason to work on your sleep hygiene is because it will help you maintain a healthy body weight, which can also play a part in controlling your condition. Although researchers aren't yet sure why, sleep deprivation seems to make you hungrier by affecting leptin and ghrelin, two hormones that regulate appetite.

Recent research has even demonstrated that you don't need to lose sleep on a regular basis to feel these effects. A small European study published in the *Journal of Sleep Research* in 2008 found that ghrelin levels and feelings of hunger were increased in nine men after only one night of poor sleep.

Data from a larger project, called the Nurses' Health Study, illustrates what can happen when people experience poor sleep over a long period of time. After following 59,813 women for 16 years, researchers found that participants who slept less than 7 hours a night were up to 32 percent more likely to have gained 15 kg (33 lbs).

So making sure you get enough sleep can become an important part of managing your psoriasis (see More Detail box on page 134).

Getting a Good Night's Sleep [MORE DETAIL]

If you're having trouble getting to sleep or staying asleep, here are a few do's and don'ts that may help you get the rest you need:

Do	Don't
Do follow a sleep schedule—go to bed around the same time every night and get up around the same time every morning	Don't stay up or sleep in too late on weekends, or you risk throwing off your sleep schedule
Do quiet, low-stress activities before bed, such as reading for pleasure, stretching, taking a warm bath, meditating or spending quiet time with a member of your household	Don't watch TV, listen to the radio, exercise or do work right before going to bed— doing things that engage your brain actively may prevent you from winding down and falling asleep
Do eat a small snack an hour or two before bed if you're hungry in the evening—try to choose foods that are high in the amino acid tryptophan (e.g., chicken, turkey, bananas, dairy products, oatmeal, eggs, fish), which can help make you sleepy	Don't consume anything containing alcohol, caffeine or refined sugar, and avoid eating large meals or drinking large amounts of fluid right before bed— they'll prevent you from falling asleep and staying asleep
Do make sure the room you're sleeping in is dark and quiet	Don't try to fall asleep listening to music, the radio or the TV, or in a room that's partially lit
Do write down anything that's on your mind—sometimes journaling your thoughts can help you stop worrying and allow you to fall asleep more easily	Don't lie awake worrying about your problems— instead, try to set them aside and think positive thoughts or write a list of things you're grateful for

Continued...

Getting a Good Night's Sleep (cont.) [MORE DETAIL]

Do	Don't
Do your best to make sure you are as physically comfortable as possible before going to bed—try adjusting the temperature of your room, applying moisturizer, taking Benadryl (diphenhydramine) if your doctor says it's okay, or taking pain medication that your doctor has prescribed	Don't go to bed too hot or cold, itchy or in pain if you can help it

Eat Healthy Food

Eating nutritious food is a sensible lifestyle choice no matter who you are—the medical community agrees that eating right is one of the best things you can do for your health. Some studies even show that what you eat can not only improve your overall well-being, but also affect your psoriasis and its treatments. We discuss these interesting and important connections in Chapter 10, so we encourage you to take some time to read that chapter—you'll learn more about how diet can play a part in influencing your disease and find out practical tips on how to fit healthy eating into your busy schedule.

"I make a very big effort to be strong, to eat healthy and to have a proper lifestyle."

ANONYMOUS PATIENT

It Doesn't Hurt to Laugh

As you deal with the ups and downs of your psoriasis, it's to be expected that you might sometimes feel depressed or anxious—and grieving is a very normal part of coming to terms with your condition. We also realize that it's hard to laugh and smile when you're in pain or itchy. But finding opportunities to have fun when you get the chance will make you feel better (see A Word from Jenny box).

> "Sometimes it's hard to have a sense of humor but you do have to have [one]."
>
> MARGIE

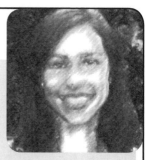

A Word from Jenny

Finding a Balance

My celiac disease flares just like psoriasis – sometimes it's well controlled and sometimes it's not (see my story on page 156). The summer of 2006 it got worse during a period of intense stress and my immunity weakened because I wasn't digesting food properly. I got pneumonia and sinusitis, and I was left feeling physically weak and emotionally drained.

The reason I had gotten sick was simple: too much work and not enough play. But changing the way I balanced my job, family commitments, socialization and household chores didn't seem simple at all. I didn't have the energy to come up with a fancy plan, so I just started letting some of my chores slide (after all, how clean did my apartment need to be?) and carving out more time for fun. I said "yes" to any party or fun outing I was invited to—even if I didn't feel like going—and laughed a lot.

At first I didn't feel happier, but after a few weeks of sticking to my new schedule, I started to feel better. To this day, I use this strategy to maintain balance in my life any time I start to feel stressed.

Quit Smoking and Drinking Alcohol

Smoking and drinking alcohol may actually make your psoriasis worse in addition to raising your risk of developing cancer and heart disease. In fact, if you smoke more than 20 cigarettes a day, you not only have a greater risk of developing cardiovascular disease, but are also more than twice as likely to have severe psoriasis, compared to non-smokers.

Although more studies will be needed before we know for sure whether smoking and drinking contribute to making psoriasis worse—or are responsible for bringing it on in the first place—the medical community agrees that avoiding smoking and excessive drinking are two of the safest and healthiest things you can do to improve your overall health. For more information on the links between smoking, drinking and psoriasis, see page 200.

"The first couple of drinks make you feel euphoric, but it's the third drink that starts the itching."

ANONYMOUS PATIENT

Chapter 10

nutrition and psoriasis

What Happens in This Chapter
- The importance of diet
- What to eat and what not to eat
- Tips on how to start making changes to your diet

Although there isn't a lot of scientific evidence showing that diet can affect psoriasis, it's still important to eat nutritious food. Eating well can help control some of the other conditions that travel with psoriasis, and it can help you feel better overall—physically, emotionally and mentally. The good news is that cooking healthily doesn't have to be time-consuming or difficult, and you don't have to give up all of your favorite dishes. A few changes here and there can sometimes make all of the difference!

Introduction

Food is central to your physical health—it can keep you strong and healthy or make you sick. Food also affects you emotionally. Digging into a big bowl of ice cream, that huge plate of spaghetti or your favorite Sunday night dinner can bring you comfort and satisfaction like nothing else. That's why modifying your diet can be very challenging.

But don't feel discouraged, especially if you've found it hard in the past to change what you eat—this chapter will give you practical tips for eating healthily and will show you that it's easier than you might think. Nutritious food can taste just as sinful as your favorite junk foods and doesn't have to involve long, complicated marathons in the kitchen.

The Connection Between Diet and Psoriasis: A Complicated Picture

Most of us are aware that eating nutritious food is important for overall health. In addition, many people with medical conditions are able to manage their diseases with diet. For example, migraine sufferers avoid headaches by staying away from certain foods. People with high cholesterol can lower their LDL ("bad cholesterol") levels by reducing their intake of trans and saturated fats.

However, the connection between diet and psoriasis is less clear. A few studies suggest that changing the foods you eat could improve your skin, but as we discussed in Chapter 9, there isn't any strong scientific evidence to support claims that specific foods influence psoriasis. Alcohol seems to be the only dietary factor that can directly affect psoriasis (see page 200)—the more you drink, the more your psoriasis may flare.

On the other hand, if you have psoriasis it's worth taking a look at what you eat for several reasons.

Perhaps the best reason is that eating right may help you avoid or manage several of the most troubling conditions that tend to travel with psoriasis, such as cardiovascular disease, diabetes and metabolic syndrome (see page 27). There are also other reasons, discussed below.

The Body Weight Connection

Eating too much generally may make your psoriasis worse. People who are obese tend to have psoriasis that is more resistant to treatment. It's not clear whether their extra weight is somehow making their psoriasis respond poorly

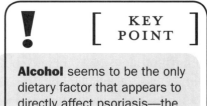

KEY POINT

Alcohol seems to be the only dietary factor that appears to directly affect psoriasis—the more you drink, the more your psoriasis may flare.

to treatment or whether their weight gain happens because severe psoriasis reduces their motivation to exercise and eat well. One factor could be inflammation (see page 30). There is some evidence to support the idea that body fat, particularly excess body fat, leads to an increase in inflammation elsewhere in the body. More research is needed to fully understand this connection.

On the other end of the scale, eating too little can also affect psoriasis, probably by suppressing the immune system. This phenomenon was accidentally discovered during World War II, when starving Dutch prisoners with psoriasis found that their skin improved.

Self-starvation is definitely not recommended as a way to improve your own psoriasis. However, some studies suggest that if you are overweight a little healthy weight loss could lead to improvements in your condition (see A Word from Dr. Papp box on next page).

A Word from Dr. Papp

A Word About Diet and Psoriasis

In the last few years, studies have shown that overweight people don't respond as well to psoriasis treatment as thin people. The reason this matters is that many people with psoriasis are overweight. Researchers think that this happens because drug doses are set for people who fall into more normal weight ranges and people who are overweight or obese need more medication before a drug will work properly for them. Heavier people may also suffer from worse psoriasis. And it's not just psoriasis. Diabetes, high blood pressure, high cholesterol and heart disease are all made worse by being overweight.

There is abundant evidence that a healthy diet leads to a longer and better life, which, in the end, can give you a greater chance of controlling your condition. I have observed after many years of practice as a dermatologist that people who eat healthily and live healthy lifestyles feel better physically, mentally and emotionally.

What About Vegan Diets?

There is a lot of debate around the benefits of **vegan** diets for people with psoriasis. Vegans avoid foods that come from animals, including eggs, honey and milk, so a vegan diet tends to be very low in "bad" fats and high in fiber. Many alternative healthcare practitioners suggest that vegan diets can reduce inflammation in the body and help reduce psoriasis symptoms; however, so far there are no solid studies to back this up.

If you are tempted to try a vegan diet, a few words of warning. Vegan diets are hard to maintain and tend to lack some key nutrients. To stay healthy while practicing a vegan diet, you need to combine grains with legumes to get enough protein. You also need to take iron and B12 supplements because the best sources for these nutrients are meat. So even if vegan diets prove to be helpful in psoriasis, many people would find it difficult to maintain this eating style.

Gluten and Psoriasis

Another much-debated link between diet and psoriasis concerns gluten, the protein found in some grains that makes people with celiac disease sick when they eat it. When doctors started noticing that some people with celiac disease and psoriasis showed improvements in both of their conditions on a gluten-free diet, more formal research was conducted.

A series of studies from Sweden suggested that if you have gliadin antibodies in your blood (an indication of celiac disease), you may see an improvement in your psoriasis if you go on a gluten-free diet. However, these studies are hard to interpret because celiac disease itself can cause skin symptoms that look like psoriasis (see Jenny's story on page 156). One thing is certain: more research needs to be conducted before we can draw any real conclusions about the connections between gluten and psoriasis.

For more on the claims around supplements, dietary factors and psoriasis, see Chapter 9.

The Bottom Line on the Diet Connection

It's important to keep in mind that the research on the effects of diet on psoriasis is in very early stages. Scientists need to conduct more studies to fully understand how and why different eating styles might affect this condition before we can start to make definite conclusions about the psoriasis-diet connection.

What to Eat

Even if the research hasn't made it clear yet whether or not eating nutritious food will affect your psoriasis, you can be sure that it will make a difference to your overall health. And the healthier you are, the stronger you'll be, the more energy you'll have and the easier it will be to accomplish the things you want to in life. In this section you'll learn about healthy eating basics and get practical tips on how to incorporate nutritious food into your busy lifestyle.

Keep It Simple

There are so many eating guidelines out there that it's hard to make sense of them all. On top of that, the rules have changed over the last few decades. The 1980s were the days of zero-fat diets, which we now know are bad for you. The 1990s marked the start of the low-carbohydrate craze. Fortunately, the new millennium has brought with it more balance and common sense.

Many of today's top nutrition professionals are advocating a simpler approach to healthy eating. They suggest a variety of whole, natural foods, most of which should be plants, such as grains, nuts, legumes, seeds, fruits and vegetables. It sounds straightforward, but these days so many processed items litter grocery store shelves that it's hard to tell what's healthy and what's not.

The best way to find nutritious foods is to learn how to read labels and adjust how you grocery shop (see How to Shop on page 146). It takes a bit of practice, but after a few weeks of shopping, choosing foods that are truly nourishing will come automatically to you.

When to Eat

It can be hard to fit eating into your busy schedule, but going hungry or skipping meals regularly isn't a good idea—you can lose energy and mental focus, and could actually gain weight. The best guideline for when to have a meal or snack is when you're hungry enough to eat, but aren't starving.

However, if you find that your sense of hunger is "off" (i.e., you're rarely hungry or are hungry all the time), you can help your body regulate itself by planning regular mealtimes and choosing the right kinds of foods. A dietitian or nutritionist can help you figure out an eating plan that works well with your schedule and food preferences.

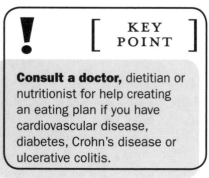

[KEY POINT]

Consult a doctor, dietitian or nutritionist for help creating an eating plan if you have cardiovascular disease, diabetes, Crohn's disease or ulcerative colitis.

How Much to Eat

You should eat until you're satisfied, but not over-stuffed and feeling sick—keep in mind that your stomach is only about the size of your fist! Also, it takes about 20 minutes for your brain to register that your stomach is full. So if you eat what's on your plate and don't immediately feel completely satisfied, wait a few minutes before deciding if you'd like seconds. The amount you eat will probably vary from day to day, depending on how physically active you've been, your individual physiology, how long you've been awake, your stress levels and the sorts of foods you're eating.

The Importance of Fat

Fat was once treated as the enemy in the world of nutrition, but we now know that fats play several critical roles in your body. "Good" fats regulate inflammation, lower cholesterol and reduce your risk of developing cardiovascular disease. Fats are also important for the proper functioning of your immune system, processing fat-soluble vitamins (i.e., A, D, E and K) and controlling body temperature. Fats are also crucial building blocks for hormones and nerves.

Canadian dietary guidelines recommend that you have 2 to 3 tbs (30 to 40 mL) of unsaturated fat a day and that you limit your total fat intake to 30 percent or less of your daily calories.

Key Ingredients

Taking a multivitamin or other nutrient supplements—even good-quality ones—won't compensate for a poor diet. Also, they could interact with your prescription medication. It's best to get all or most of your vitamins, minerals and essential fats from the food you eat. Here are a few key ingredients that can help you stay as healthy as possible as you deal with the ups and downs of your psoriasis:

- **Water**: Drinking plenty of water can help you keep your energy up and weight in check.
- **Fresh fruits and vegetables**: These foods are packed with vitamins, minerals and antioxidants to help heal your skin and regulate your immunity. Eat a rainbow (i.e., many different colors) of fruits and vegetables every day to ensure you're getting a variety of nutrients.
- **Nuts, seeds and legumes**: These foods are full of fiber and healthy plant protein that will help satisfy your hunger and prevent unhealthy snacking. Nuts and seeds also contain cholesterol-lowering, anti-inflammatory "good" fat. Some (e.g., sesame seeds, almonds) are good sources of calcium.

- **Whole grains:** The nutrients and fiber in whole grains such as whole wheat, brown rice, whole oats, quinoa, millet, buckwheat and barley can help keep your bowels regular and manage high cholesterol.
- **Meat and fish:** Lean meat can be a healthy part of your diet. Aim for a portion about the size of your palm (no larger). Oily fish, such as salmon, mackerel, trout, herring and sardines, are excellent sources of cholesterol-lowering, anti-inflammatory "good" fat. If you're worried about the mercury levels in fish, find out which kinds are safest by visiting the Environmental Defense Fund's Seafood Selector website listed in the Resources section of this book.

How to Shop

How you shop for groceries has a huge effect on what you eat. Here are a few guidelines on how to make your trips to the supermarket stress-free:

- Make a shopping list before you go. If you're disorganized, you'll waste time wandering aimlessly and spend money on food you may not need.
- Don't shop when you're hungry. If you do, you'll probably buy too much food and products that aren't healthy.
- Read labels before you buy anything in a package. Make sure the ingredients are all real, whole, natural foods (e.g., nuts, fruit, eggs) and that the product doesn't have too much sugar, "bad" fat or salt. A quick way to determine whether the item contains unprocessed ingredients is to look at the expiry date: check that it expires within days, weeks or months, not years.

- Aim to buy food that is mostly located around the periphery of the grocery store—fresh or frozen fruits and vegetables, eggs, unprocessed meats and dairy. The only sorts of items you might need to get from the aisles include nuts, legumes, seeds and whole grains.

Other Weight Loss Tips

Aside from eating whole, natural foods and having a well-planned shopping strategy, there are a few other tricks to losing weight. Below is a list of do's and don'ts that might help you shed extra pounds:

Do	Don't
Do eat foods high in fiber and "good" fats—they help lower your cholesterol and keep you full so you aren't tempted to eat unhealthy snacks.	**Don't let stress get to you**—chronic stress can lead to weight gain because your body releases cortisol, a hormone that can actually make you hungrier (see Chapter 11 for stress—reduction techniques).
Do exercise—exercising is good for your immune system; it burns calories, boosts your energy and helps your body circulate nutrients and oxygen.	**Don't starve yourself**—going on a low-calorie diet isn't sustainable and trains your body to function on less food. When you finally go off the diet, you will gain even more weight.
Do cook—it doesn't have to take long, but it's the best way to control your portion sizes and the ingredients in your food (see A Word From Jenny on page 149).	**Don't try to lose more than 1 pound a week**—healthy, gradual weight loss increases your chances of keeping the pounds off.

Continued...

Do	Don't
Do drink plenty of water—other drinks tend to have "empty" calories, sugar or synthetic chemicals. Water is also cheap—it will help fill you up and boost your energy if you're dehydrated. You know you're hydrated enough if your urine is very light yellow. Also keep in mind that sometimes thirst is mistaken for hunger. Next time you're hungry, try drinking some water before reaching for food.	**Don't keep junk food in your home or at the office**—if it's not there, you can't eat it!
Do use smaller plates—if your plates are smaller, you'll eat less. If you don't want to invest in new dishes, eat your main meals off your snack or salad plates.	**Don't eat straight out of the container**—it will help prevent bingeing. If you want a snack, try putting a handful of the food you want in a bowl or on a plate before you start to eat it. That way you won't end up eating more than one portion!
Do try starting your meal with a salad—it will fill you up a bit before you start eating the heavier part of your meal, such as meat or pasta.	**Don't consume too much caffeine**—it can stay in your system for several hours, which can disrupt your sleep. Not sleeping enough is directly linked to weight gain (see Get Enough Sleep on page 132).

A Word from Jenny

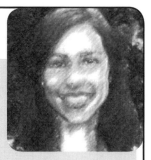

Finding Time to Cook

One of the best ways to maintain a healthy weight is to cook. Unfortunately, in our fast-food world, we've been tricked into believing that cooking from scratch is too hard and time-consuming. This simply isn't true. I cook almost everything I eat from scratch because I have celiac disease (see my story on page 156). I can whip up the most mouth-watering, simple dishes in the same (or less) amount of time it takes to grab fast food or wait for a pizza delivery.

My secret to success is keeping it simple and planning my meals. I start by taking a few minutes once a week to figure out what I want to eat, and I look in my fridge and cupboards to see what I already have and what I still need. Then I schedule specific times to pick up groceries and cook.

I spend very little time in the kitchen because my recipes are easy and made of everyday ingredients (visit www.yourpsoriasis.org for some of my favorite dishes). If I make a meal that's a bit more labor-intensive, I shop one day, prepare my ingredients (e.g., chop vegetables, mix spices) the next and cook the day after. This way, it doesn't feel like such a big job.

I always make large batches of food and live off the leftovers, which means I don't cook often. If I really can't find time to cook, I make smart take-out choices, such as a pre-cooked chicken from the deli counter of my grocery store and a large, simple salad. And I keep my snacks really straightforward. I turn to whole, natural foods because it takes no time to grab an apple, a handful of nuts or some pre-chopped vegetables.

What Not to Eat

Just as the rules guiding what you should eat are relatively simple, so are the rules for what you shouldn't eat—try to avoid processed and packaged foods filled with ingredients that you aren't familiar with or can't pronounce.

The reason that most processed products are so bad for you is that they tend to be low in nutrition. Even if the pre-packaged food you're eating has enough calories to keep you going, it may not have enough vitamins, minerals and other nutrients (e.g., "good" fats) to allow your body to function at its best, especially over the long-term.

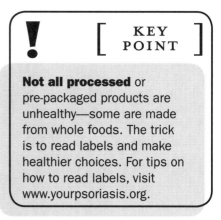

! [**KEY POINT**]

Not all processed or pre-packaged products are unhealthy—some are made from whole foods. The trick is to read labels and make healthier choices. For tips on how to read labels, visit www.yourpsoriasis.org.

Many processed foods are also extremely high in trans fat, sugar and salt, which are unhealthy and trick your taste buds into thinking that nutritious whole foods are bland and impossible to enjoy. And beware of products that claim to be "fortified"—they've had most of their nutrients removed through processing and usually only a tiny amount of artificially created vitamins and minerals have been added back in.

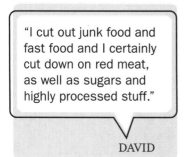

"I cut out junk food and fast food and I certainly cut down on red meat, as well as sugars and highly processed stuff."

DAVID

It's important to avoid deep-fried foods, as well, because they can be extremely high in fat. And if you have diabetes or high cholesterol, you may want to limit how many eggs you eat. Although the large amount of cholesterol in eggs doesn't normally affect blood cholesterol levels, people with diabetes and high cholesterol can be more sensitive to it.

It's also a good idea for all of us to reduce how much meat we eat— you can start by enjoying one meat-free meal a week. Or be daring and try "meatless Mondays," a wise suggestion from food writer Michael Pollan.

Finally, try not to over-sweeten your food when you're cooking or baking from scratch. If you want to add sweetness, it's best to use small amounts of the most natural sources of sugar you can find. Raw and unpasteurized honey is a natural source of sugar (note that children under age 1 shouldn't eat honey because of the risk of getting a bacterial infection called botulism). Another source is fruit, such as unsweetened applesauce, chopped dates or mashed bananas. These more natural ways to sweeten food have nutritional value—they can help you feel fuller and more satisfied, and prevent unhealthy snacking.

Pure maple syrup and molasses are other possibilities, even though they are processed, because they have more nutrients than refined white sugar, brown sugar, corn syrup and high-fructose corn syrup. However, these highly caloric natural products remain simple sugars. They can still cause the same problems as processed sweeteners with no nutritional value if you eat too much of them. The secret is always moderation!

See What to Eat on page 143 for tips on how to choose healthy foods, and visit www.yourpsoriasis.org for soul-satisfying dishes that are quick and nutritious.

Making Dietary Changes:
One Step at a Time

Everyone takes a different amount of time and a different approach, but most people prefer to modify their diet slowly. So try replacing one unhealthy habit at a time and be patient with yourself—change is hard.

Start by cutting back on the number of soft drinks, and choose one day a week to enjoy a home-cooked dinner. Or add a piece of fruit to each of your meals. Keeping a food log is a great way to help you identify some of your eating patterns, which can make it easier for you to modify them and track your progress—you might even start to notice a connection between your flares and certain foods.

And if you're feeling lost or frustrated, you can always consult a nutritionist or dietitian (see the Resources section at the back of this book for ways to find a nutrition professional). Above all, remember that every change counts, no matter how small!

"I still eat everything everybody else eats, but I eat smaller portions. I tell you it works—and it's not like a 'diet.' As time goes on it gets easier because...my body's getting used to not eating big meals. It's really good and you feel better...now I've got my [blood] sugar under control."

TOM
(WHO HAS DIABETES)

Chapter **11**

overcoming emotional challenges

What Happens in This Chapter
- What you and your loved ones might be feeling and why
- Talking to others about your psoriasis
- How to form a support network
- Knowing when to seek professional counseling
- How to make yourself feel better
- Tips for your loved ones

Psoriasis can affect your emotions as much as it affects your skin. It's normal to feel sad or scared as you go through the ups and downs of your condition, but there are ways to overcome negative emotions. Forming a strong support network, learning how to reduce your stress and knowing the best way to talk to others about your psoriasis can go a long way toward helping you get the most out of life. Lots of people with this condition enjoy happy, fulfilled lives, and so can you.

Introduction

If you're feeling like your psoriasis is getting you down and you're not sure how to help yourself feel better, this chapter is for you. We'll guide you through the emotional journey that often accompanies psoriasis so you can understand why you're feeling the way you are and learn how to deal with your emotions in a healthy way. You'll also read practical tips on how to overcome some of the social challenges you may face as you live with your condition.

Whatever You're Feeling Is Normal

You might be experiencing many emotions right now, and it's important to know that all of them are normal. Whether you're sad, angry, anxious or shocked, it's okay. Although the inflammation in your body could be contributing to feelings of depression (see page 25), your mind is trying to adjust to something new and upsetting—a change in your health and appearance. You are, at some level, grieving.

Many of us think that grief only happens when someone dies, but this isn't true. We can grieve any loss, including the loss of a job, a house, a relationship, our health or the health of a loved one. In her 1969 book *On Death and Dying*, Elisabeth Kübler-Ross outlined five stages of grief that many people experience when they suffer a loss— you might be able to relate to some of them:

1. **Denial:** At first, you might feel lost and shocked, and unable to believe what's happening. Denial is your mind's way of protecting you from being overwhelmed by emotions.
2. **Anger:** Many people are afraid to feel angry, but allowing yourself to be mad will start to open the door to overcoming your loss. You might be mad at your friends, your family, your doctors or God.

3. **Bargaining**: At some point, you might wish that psoriasis had never happened to you, and you might ask for it to go away. You may find yourself negotiating with God or your doctors.

4. **Depression**: Once reality starts to set in and you begin to accept your loss, you may feel depressed. It may seem like your sadness will never end, but you will eventually feel better.

5. **Acceptance**: This stage is about accepting the reality of your new situation. It doesn't necessarily mean that you're okay with having psoriasis—although you might be having more good days than bad at this point—but it is a sign that you're on your way to letting psoriasis become a part of your life, rather than seeing it as an unwanted intrusion.

It's important to understand that emotions don't fit into neat and tidy packages. Every loss is different, as is every person who suffers a loss. So it's typical to skip or repeat some of these stages, or experience them in a different order. Nevertheless, knowing about them might help you make some sense of what you're going through. It's also important to know that there is no time limit on grief.

Keep in mind, as well, that you may not be the only one who is feeling upset. It's common for the people closest to you to have a hard time accepting your psoriasis diagnosis, and they could also experience some of the stages of grief. In addition, they could be holding some of their feelings back because they are afraid to express them or unsure how to start a conversation about them.

> "It affected me—people looking at you, even going to somebody's house and you sit in their chair. You get up and you can see where the psoriasis has fallen off. It's embarrassing."
>
> TOM

A Word from Jenny

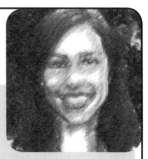

Facing Life Challenges

It's easy to feel overwhelmed when you have a disease, especially when you're first diagnosed or if your condition suddenly becomes worse. I know—I have celiac disease. I remember when I became sick. I had chronic diarrhea and strange skin problems, including rashes that scarred me, and toes that were so itchy I'd wake up from a dead sleep already scratching them. I started to worry about whether I'd be able to live a productive life or whether someone would want to date or marry me.

When we finally figured out what was wrong and I realized that I had to change my entire diet, I was afraid that I'd never enjoy eating again and that life would be a constant burden. I had food dreams night after night and questioned whether I would ever feel happy. Now, all that trauma seems very far away. My skin stays calm as long as I avoid certain foods, and I don't even think about what I eat. It's just automatic for me to cook everything from scratch (visit www.yourpsoriasis.org for some of my healthy, simple, delicious recipes).

I also realized that everyone I know has at some point faced a health issue or major challenge that has made them stop and ask, "Will this ruin my life?" Going through and overcoming hard times is normal. What's important is that you develop coping mechanisms and keep putting one foot in front of the other. Eventually, you will create a new life balance and you might even find renewed purpose as an activist, educator or mentor for others in your community.

Talking to Others About Your Disease

It's hard enough having psoriasis, but it can be even harder when you're forced to explain why your skin looks the way it does to people who ask questions or make rude comments about your appearance, such as:

- "What's wrong with your skin?"
- "Are you okay?"
- "Don't touch me."
- "Can I touch you?"
- "Is that contagious?"
- "How did you get that?"
- "You can't be here/touch that/use that."

> "You have to forgive yourself for having it, and you have to forget the suffering you went through and learn from it."
>
> ANONYMOUS PATIENT

Although it's hard not to take statements like this personally, know that people usually say something because they're concerned, scared, surprised or curious. They very rarely mean to hurt or offend you. The best way to deal with these situations is to be factual and straightforward.

Try something like, "I have a disease called psoriasis. I've had it for many years and it's not contagious." You then might be asked follow-up questions, and this is your chance to educate whomever you're talking to. If it becomes obvious that the person you're dealing with is trying to be cruel, simply ignore him or her—that's the only effective way to handle a bully.

> "I just kind of coped with it. It was tough. If somebody doesn't like me because I've got it, that's life. It's not my fault."
>
> TOM

To make sure you feel prepared to deal with being approached by strangers, practice how you might respond to different questions. Talk to your

> "It's surprising that when you actually bring it out into the open with some people, how many people out there say 'my mom has that' or 'my brother has that' or 'my cousin has that,' and it's not the first time they've seen somebody in that situation."
>
> CHRIS

reflection in a mirror, into your computer microphone or to a loved one until you are comfortable with what you want to say. The calmer and more relaxed you are about describing your disease, the more accepting others will be of it. People around you will take your lead, so if it's no big deal to you, it will be no big deal to them. You might also be surprised at how many people will share their own health-related stories with you!

Talking to a Date or Partner

There's no reason to talk about your psoriasis on a first date. If you are tempted to mention your condition, ask yourself why you feel compelled to say something—if you're doing it because you feel regretful or are seeking forgiveness, skip it. If your date has a problem with your psoriasis, then he or she isn't the right person for you. Cross that person off your list and move on!

If you want to tell your potential partner because he or she has specifically brought up the subject of psoriasis in conversation, has asked about the appearance of your skin, or is about to see you with your clothes off for the first time, then you can feel free to provide a short and simple explanation that is factual, relaxed and non-apologetic. The same thing goes if you're about to discuss marriage and the genetic implications of psoriasis.

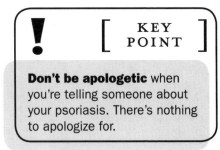

! **[KEY POINT]**

Don't be apologetic when you're telling someone about your psoriasis. There's nothing to apologize for.

If you're already married or seriously dating someone when you're diagnosed with psoriasis, you'll have to work together to keep communicating and compromising. Be open with your partner about your fears and feelings. Talk about how your day-to-day routines and long-term goals may need to change. Bringing issues like these into the open can be a relief for both of you and is an important step toward finding a new rhythm as a couple. Set aside a time to discuss what's on your mind when you're not rushed or tired, and write down what you want to say first so your thoughts are clear. Avoid using accusatory or defensive language by starting your statements with "I" instead of "you," and try the active listening technique described on page 168.

> "I had some flack with my wife because of the mess it made. It does involve your personal life. It's a matter of doing the best you can do and it all works out."
>
> TOM

Handling "The Look"

People you encounter may also give you disapproving looks. There's not a whole lot you can do if that happens. You can try flashing a smile, which often neutralizes a funny glance (it's much harder to be rude to or judge someone who's friendly), or you can simply ignore the situation.

It's important to realize that you can't control others; you can only control your actions and feelings. If someone doesn't approve of what you look like, that's their problem, not yours! Do your best not to let others' opinions bother you—remember that they're reacting to something superficial and not to the real you.

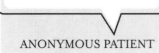

"People rarely will say anything, but you get 'the look.' How are you supposed to react to a look? What are you supposed to say? There are no one-liners."

ANONYMOUS PATIENT

Although psoriasis attacks your identity by changing your appearance, it's important to remember that your value as a person is not determined by what you look like. Don't let your psoriasis define you, and know that you're perfect just the way you are. See How to Help Yourself Feel Better on page 163 for tips on how to boost your self-esteem and confidence.

Forming a Support Network

As we mentioned in Chapter 5, it's important to have a support network as you go through your psoriasis journey. There are lots of ways to expand your group of friends so you'll have more people to both laugh and cry with. You can also seek more formal kinds of support, such as counseling, if that suits you better.

- **Eat with other people**: People used to eat communally all the time, whereas nowadays we eat alone, in meetings or on the run. But sharing mealtime with friends and family is a great way to lift your spirits. Host a dinner party or potluck and get introduced to new people by asking your friends to bring someone you've never met. Visit www.yourpsoriasis.org for recipe ideas.

- **Spend quality time with your family**: Nowadays, many families are so busy that they don't spend a lot of time together. However, there are ways of reconnecting with your family to make them a key part of your support network. Turn off your TVs and computers, and play a board game, go for a walk, go to the museum, play in the park or take a road trip together. Find ways to talk, laugh, share and bond.

- **Take up a hobby:** One of the best ways to connect with others is to participate in activities that you enjoy. You might want to join a sports team, hiking club, choir, church or synagogue group, or chess club. You can take dance classes, photography lessons or learn a new language. Any kind of structured group activity will do.
- **Say "yes":** If you get invited somewhere, such as a party, say yes, even if you don't know anyone. What's the worst that could happen? If you find that you aren't connecting with anyone there, you can leave early. You never know who you might meet.
- **Join a community center:** Joining your local community center will help introduce you to others in your neighborhood and give you a regular place to go to learn new skills and socialize.
- **Join a support group:** Even if you can't find a support group specifically for people with psoriasis, you can attend meetings for people overcoming similar life challenges, such as stress, anger or depression.
- **Speak with a mental health professional:** Another way to get support, particularly if you find that talking to loved ones isn't helpful, is to consult a mental health professional, such as a social worker, psychiatrist, psychotherapist, psychologist, therapist or counselor—anyone with professional training in helping people through rough times will do!

If you're used to working a lot and don't socialize much, you need to understand that learning to form connections with others takes time and practice. Keep reaching out until you find what works for you, and, before you know it, you'll feel much less alone.

> "Just tell people exactly what's going on and it helps. All my close friends, they all understood, and it was never an issue with them after I explained what it was."
>
> TOM

When to Seek Professional Counseling

It makes sense to feel upset as you adjust to life with psoriasis. However, there might come a point when you're feeling so bad that you wonder whether you should seek professional counseling. The reality is that everyone's needs are different, and you have to decide for yourself whether you're ready for a therapy referral. Experts usually recommend that you seek professional assistance if:

- You feel you want to talk to a therapist
- You feel you don't know how to handle your emotions
- You want help in reducing your stress levels
- You're having frequent and very dark thoughts (e.g., thoughts of suicide, fear and hopelessness)
- Your ability to function normally has been disrupted (e.g., you're having trouble eating, sleeping, socializing and concentrating at work)
- Your sex drive has decreased
- Your mood has changed (e.g., you cry a lot and can't seem to cheer up, or you're angry all the time)

You can ask your family doctor for a referral to a therapist, or you can find one through the Resources section at the back of this book.

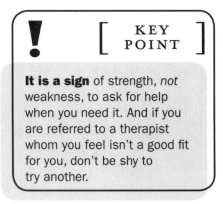

! [KEY POINT]

It is a sign of strength, *not* weakness, to ask for help when you need it. And if you are referred to a therapist whom you feel isn't a good fit for you, don't be shy to try another.

How to Help Yourself Feel Better

It can be tempting to withdraw from the world and give up if you're going through a hard time, or shove your emotions aside and ignore them. But bad feelings are just as valid as good ones because they are a part of the healing process. What's important is that you acknowledge your feelings and deal with them in a healthy way. It's essential to keep reaching out to others, being as active as possible and caring for yourself. This section gives you a few suggestions that should help you start to work through your emotions so you can stay productive.

Minimize Negative Thoughts

Although having negative thoughts when you're stressed out is understandable, you shouldn't let them take over your life. There are exercises you can do to help process some of these thoughts and build a new perspective on how your psoriasis fits into your self-image:

- **Identify what's really bothering you:** Is it the fact that your skin looks different? Is it that you don't like the physical discomfort? Are you worried about whether you'll lose friends or your partner? Are you worried you'll never feel well again? Putting your fears into writing will allow you to address them head-on and find realistic solutions to your problems.
- **Challenge your beliefs:** Once you've identified what's bothering you, challenge any beliefs that are false. For example, if you believe that you'll never get married because of your psoriasis, it's important to realize that you can't possibly know that, so don't let that thought occupy your mind and set your mood. (By the way, all of the people with psoriasis whom we interviewed for this book are happily married.)
- **Work on accepting yourself just as you are:** Getting used to an altered appearance is one of the hardest things you might ever

have to do, but you can learn to love yourself just the way you are. Make a list of all of the things about your body that you like, surround yourself with people who love you and engage in activities that boost your confidence (see also Get Involved With the World Around You on page 165).

- **Keep a gratitude journal**: Take time first thing in the morning or before you go to bed to write down at least three things you're feeling grateful for. It can be anything—your job, the roof over your head, the sunny sky, your pet, your family, your new car. Reminding yourself about the good things in your life won't make your problems disappear, but it will help take some of the emphasis off what's upsetting you.

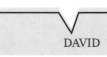

"I just sort of took things day by day and tried not to look too far down the pike, because when I did that I would get very depressed."

DAVID

Express Yourself

Keeping your emotions bottled up inside you or trying to ignore them will probably only make your stress and unhappiness worse. Try letting your feelings out—you can do this by talking to loved ones, calling a support hotline, joining a support group or consulting a therapist. If talking about your problems isn't for you, there are lots of other ways to express yourself. You can cry, scream, write down your feelings in a journal, dance creatively, take some of your anger out in a boxing class at the gym, write a song or draw a picture of your pain. Whatever type of emotional release feels right for you is just fine.

Get Involved With the World Around You

Sometimes the best thing you can do is distract yourself and take a break from worrying. Meditation is one way to keep negative thoughts at bay, but going out into the world and fully engaging in life will also do the trick. You'll meet new people, learn new skills and build self-confidence. Take up a hobby and learn how to do something you've always wanted to do; make a difference in others' lives by doing volunteer work; be a social butterfly—go to parties and organize fun outings.

Surround Yourself With Things That Make You Happy

Surrounding yourself with uplifting images and people can go a long way toward boosting your mood. Try playing with a pet or a child, or watching television shows and movies that make you feel good. Visit with family and friends who make you laugh. Spend time in your favorite places, such as a special corner of your house, or a favorite restaurant, museum or vacation spot.

Reduce Your Stress

Reducing your stress can be challenging, but with time and practice you can learn to control your anxiety and calm your mind. There are many ways to lower your stress levels and we've outlined a few of the most common ones below. If the itch or pain of your skin is too much of a distraction to successfully complete standard relaxation exercises, try asking a trained therapist or meditation instructor for advice (see the Resources section for information on how to find a skilled professional).

Meditation

Meditation is an ancient practice that was first formalized in India thousands of years ago. It can be a very powerful tool for controlling stress. It focuses and calms your mind by bringing you into the present instead of allowing you to dwell on the past or worry about the future. There are lots of different ways to meditate, but the simplest form involves sitting in an upright position with your eyes closed and paying attention only to your breath. Sounds easy, right? Give it a try and you'll find out how hard it really is!

Your mind will wander constantly at first, but by limiting these scattered thoughts, you will learn to stop negative beliefs before they turn into irrational and possibly untrue fears. To conquer your busy mind, gently guide your attention back to your breath and don't let yourself get frustrated. It takes weeks or months to be able to focus enough to really see benefits. Stick with it and you'll discover what it's like to be still and think clearly. For meditation resoures, see the back of this book.

The Power of Meditation [**MORE DETAIL**]

Jon Kabat-Zinn runs the University of Massachusetts Medical Center's Stress Reduction and Relaxation Program (SR&RP), which helps people with a wide variety of serious conditions reduce their stress levels and improve their tolerance to physical discomfort. In his book *Full Catastrophe Living*, Kabat-Zinn describes how the SR&RP participants, many of whom are at the limit of what they feel they can tolerate, are transformed by practicing meditation.

For example, one man in his seventies had such severe pain that he came to the first meditation class in a wheelchair and said that he wished he could cut off his feet. But by the end of the 8-week program, he was walking with a cane. He explained that although his pain hadn't changed much, his attitude toward it had and it seemed a lot more bearable. His wife reported that his continued commitment to meditation after the program ended was allowing him to lead a happy and active life.

Deep Breathing

Believe it or not, breathing properly can help you calm down. Deep full breaths are a powerful, yet simple way to relax. However, most of us breathe shallowly from the chest and shoulders. To change how you breathe, inhale slowly through your nose to completely fill your lungs with air, which will cause your belly, rather than your chest, to rise. Then exhale slowly through your nose (your belly should fall). You can encourage deep breathing by counting to three as you inhale and exhale.

Visualization

Another tried and true relaxation method is **visualization**. Start by sitting in a relaxed, comfortable position and breathe slowly and deeply. Then focus on a peaceful thought or imagine a beautiful place. As with meditation, your mind will probably wander—that's okay. Gently guide yourself back to your internal place of comfort and stay there for several minutes.

Progressive Muscle Relaxation

Progressive muscle relaxation can help undo some of the tension you hold in your muscles. It is generally done lying on the ground with your eyes closed and involves tensing and then relaxing each group of muscles one by one throughout your body, starting at your feet. To begin, scrunch your toes tightly for 5 to 10 seconds and then release and stretch them. Move to your ankles and then your lower legs and thighs. Keep going up your body and down your arms. When you finally get to your forehead, you're done.

Exercise

The chemicals changes in your body during a workout, combined with the sense of accomplishment you feel from socializing and learning new skills, can be a powerful tool in reducing stress and easing depression. See page 129 for more information about the benefits of exercise, tips on how to get started on an exercise program and how to overcome some of the challenges involved in exercising with psoriasis.

Tips for Your Loved Ones

Your loved ones might not be sure how to help you during this challenging time, so feel free to refer them to this section for some guidance.

How to Help a Loved One With Psoriasis

If someone close to you has just been diagnosed with psoriasis, you might be feeling a bit helpless. You might also feel sad, angry or anxious. All of these emotions are normal and are to be expected when the health of a loved one is affected. Your friend or family member is feeling many of the same emotions you are, so it's important to be there for each other.

The first thing you can do is to be empathetic by acknowledging how hard it is to struggle with an illness. Try a technique called active listening. It involves repeating in your own words what you've just heard your conversation partner say (e.g., It seems like you're feeling scared about your future because you don't know if you'll feel well enough to work; is this right?). You won't necessarily be able to provide solutions to your loved one's problems, but listening actively will show that you care and that you're there to be as supportive as possible. You should also check in with your

> "I have three sisters who never had it, and they never understood. It got to the point where no one visited me in the hospital anymore because I'd been in the hospital so many times."
>
> ANONYMOUS PATIENT

loved one from time to time and ask if everything's okay, especially if he or she seems down. Don't accept answers like "nothing" or "never mind" when you ask what's wrong—listen to your gut. If someone you care about has had a significant change in mood or behavior (e.g., a loss of appetite, sex drive, sleep, focus at work), be caring but persistent. If the problem seems serious, take the lead and suggest that your loved one seek professional counseling. It might be necessary for you to make the first appointment on his or her behalf.

> **!** **[KEY POINT]**
>
> **If someone you know** threatens suicide, call 911. Even if you're not sure whether your loved one will go through with his or her plan, it's always better to be safe than sorry. You'll never get in trouble for calling 911 if you have a legitimate reason to think that someone's life is in danger.

How to Get Support

Of course, no one should have to shoulder the burden of caring for a sick friend or family member alone. If you're feeling overwhelmed, don't be afraid to ask for help. Join a support group for caregivers, or get other friends or family members to lend a hand so you can take breaks. You can also read How to Help Yourself Feel Better on page 163 for information on how to manage your emotions. It's important to take care of yourself, or you will become burned out.

Chapter **12**

psoriasis under special circumstances

What Happens in This Chapter
- Psoriasis treatment before, during and after pregnancy
- Treating psoriasis in people over age 65
- Psoriasis treatment for people with hepatitis B or C, or HIV
- Treating psoriasis in people with cancer or who are having surgery
- Vaccinations and psoriasis treatments

If you are facing health challenges beyond your psoriasis, many treatment options are still available for you. Whether you're considering parenthood, turning 65, want to get vaccinated, are having surgery or have an illness such as hepatitis, HIV or cancer, your doctor can come up with a therapy plan that meets your needs.

Introduction

In Chapters 7 and 9, we talked about the many treatment options for psoriasis, but it's important to keep in mind that not all of these choices may be right for you. Beyond just your lifestyle and personal preferences, there could be other factors influencing the course of your disease and which treatments you are eligible to try.

In this chapter you'll learn how other special factors about your life can affect your psoriasis journey. You can find information about children and psoriasis in Chapter 13.

If You're Pregnant or Thinking About Fatherhood

Having a baby is without a doubt one of the most exciting times in your life. But it can be frustrating and scary to get sick just as you're contemplating conceiving, during pregnancy or while nursing. The good news is that despite the challenges involved in treating psoriasis before, during and after pregnancy, it is possible to gain some relief from symptoms, even without the help of medication!

If you are pregnant, planning on getting pregnant, or nursing, or if you are considering fatherhood, your first order of business should be to tell your doctor. Then we suggest asking the questions on the next page.

Questions for women to ask	Questions for men to ask
• What are my treatment options before, during and after pregnancy?	• What are my treatment options before, during and after my partner is pregnant?
• How thoroughly have these treatments been studied in pregnant and nursing women?	• How thoroughly have these treatments been studied in fathers?
• What are the benefits and drawbacks of each of these treatments? What about their potential side effects for me and my baby?	• What are the benefits and drawbacks of each of these treatments? What about their potential side effects for me and a baby?
• How long does it take for these drugs to completely leave my system?	• How long does it take for these drugs to completely leave my system?
• How might being pregnant affect my disease?	• How long do I have to wait after taking medications that can harm the baby before I can get my partner pregnant?
• How long do I have to wait after taking medications that can harm a baby before I can get pregnant?	

Treatment Before and During Pregnancy

For Women

Interestingly, pregnancy can influence psoriasis. About 15 percent of women develop psoriasis for the first time during pregnancy, or flare if they already have the condition. About 30 to 50 percent of women find that their psoriasis improves when they are pregnant, and about 30 percent notice no change. Changes in the immune system during pregnancy are thought to be responsible for this phenomenon.

According to an Icelandic study published in 2006, women who carry a certain gene (HLA-Cw*0602, which is the best known and best studied gene variant associated with psoriasis) are most likely to experience substantial improvement in their psoriasis during pregnancy. If you do find your skin clears while you're pregnant, your symptoms are, unfortunately, likely to return afterwards.

If your psoriasis is bothering you before or during your pregnancy, your physician may not change your topical care. However, he or she may take you off tazarotene, which has been linked to birth defects. To understand more about risks when choosing your drug therapy, see page 84.

If your psoriasis is more severe, your doctor may consider light therapy, cyclosporine or biologics (see pages 75, 81 and 85) to help relieve your symptoms during pregnancy. Acitretin (see page 79) and methotrexate (see page 82) won't be options for you because they may harm your baby. As with any treatment plan, you and your doctor will work together to find what is best for you.

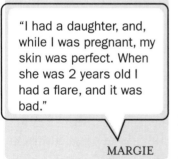

"I had a daughter, and, while I was pregnant, my skin was perfect. When she was 2 years old I had a flare, and it was bad."

MARGIE

For Men

Unfortunately, there isn't a lot of information available on how a fetus might be affected if the father, rather than the mother, is taking psoriasis medication. Methotrexate has been linked to oligospermia (a low sperm count), but there is no evidence that this side effect can damage a fetus. Although there is no strong scientific data about methotrexate and fatherhood, your doctor may take a conservative approach and ask you to use birth control if you're taking methotrexate, as well as delay attempts to conceive for at least 3 months after you stop treatment with this medication.

Methotrexate is broken down and eliminated from the body quite quickly—in a matter of days. Given that new sperm are produced in about a week, 4 weeks off methotrexate should be enough to ensure that the drug doesn't affect your sperm production.

You will certainly be asked to use birth control if you are taking acitretin. Although we know for sure that this medication causes fetal birth defects during pregnancy, we don't know whether a fetus can be harmed when the father takes it. Just to be safe, your physician will ask you to avoid conceiving during your treatment and for 3 years after you stop taking acitretin.

For Nursing Mothers

As with pregnancy, there are some psoriasis medications that you shouldn't take while you're nursing. Methotrexate and acitretin are two—they are secreted in breast milk and no studies have been done on whether or not the amount of drug passed on to the baby is safe. Your doctor will also recommend that you avoid using oral psoralen (see page 76). However, it is safe for you to use vitamin D–based medications and steroid creams, as well as undergo UVB if your disease is more severe.

If You're Over Age 65

If you have psoriasis later in life, you have many treatment options, even though you may face a few additional challenges. For example, as you age, you become more likely to experience drug-related side effects, which means that you may not be able to finish a full course of psoriasis treatment.

In addition, psoriasis drugs that can damage your liver or that your body eliminates through your kidneys, such as methotrexate (see page 82), need to be used with caution or prescribed in smaller doses. Certain psoriasis medications may also be completely off limits if you have other conditions, such as high blood pressure, or if you are taking other drugs.

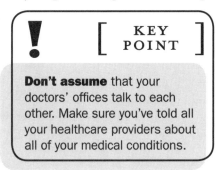

[KEY POINT]

Most older people with psoriasis have had it for much of their lives, but it is possible to develop psoriasis for the first time over the age of 65.

Topical Treatments

Topical medications are often your doctor's first line of attack because they tend to be safer and more easily tolerated by people over the age of 65. One of the most effective and best-tolerated topicals for people of all ages is Dovobet, a combination vitamin D-steroid ointment (see page 95).

Biologic Treatments

There are two biologic drugs that your doctor might prescribe if your psoriasis isn't controlled with a topical treatment. Alefacept and etanercept (see pages 92 and 89) have both been studied in people who have psoriasis later in life and have been found to be just as effective and safe in older people.

Light Therapy

Although light therapy, or phototherapy, hasn't been studied much in people over age 65, physicians still consider it a potentially valuable option for relieving symptoms. For example, a Swedish study on postmenopausal women published in 2007 found that treating them with UVB two to three times a week for 8 to 12 weeks successfully controlled their plaque psoriasis. This is similar to results in other groups of people with psoriasis.

[KEY POINT]

Don't assume that your doctors' offices talk to each other. Make sure you've told all your healthcare providers about all of your medical conditions.

If You Have Hepatitis B or C

If you have hepatitis B or C, your psoriasis treatment options will be limited, because some medications aren't appropriate for you. However, there are still many ways to relieve your symptoms. Although methotrexate isn't a good choice, other topical treatments are considered your safest option because some systemic therapies can further damage your liver or even reactivate your hepatitis. There are also some systemic medications that your doctor may consider prescribing if your psoriasis isn't getting better with a topical treatment.

Systemic Treatment in Hepatitis B

The only drug that's truly off limits if you have hepatitis B is methotrexate (see page 82), because it can cause liver damage. You may be eligible to take biologic drugs (see page 85), even though they have been known to cause hepatitis to return in some people and may have been responsible for liver complications in people with active hepatitis B.

If your doctor decides to put you on a TNF-antagonist such as etanercept, adalimumab or infliximab, you will have to take an antinucleotide hepatitis B drug to prevent your hepatitis B infection from becoming worse. If you are a candidate for biologic therapy and your hepatitis is inactive, you will be given antiviral medication 2 to 4 weeks before starting a biologic drug. Your doctor will then closely monitor your liver function and viral load while you are on this medication.

Systemic Treatment in Hepatitis C

There isn't much information on systemic treatments in people with hepatitis C. However, the limited findings to date suggest that it may be safe for you to take biologic drugs if you are carefully monitored. If your doctor thinks that you might need to take biologic medication over a long period of time, you may be sent for a liver biopsy before starting treatment.

Cyclosporine is another treatment option for you if you have hepatitis C, because it appears to have the potential to both clear up psoriasis and suppress the replication of the hepatitis C virus.

> *Hepatitis Risk and Psoriasis* [**MORE DETAIL**]
>
> People with psoriasis and other conditions that cause the skin to break have an increased risk of catching hepatitis B or C through contact with infected bodily fluids. This is one of the many reasons it is important to get your condition under control.

If You Have HIV

HIV-associated psoriasis tends to be more severe, harder to treat and more frequently accompanied by arthritis. However, psoriasis and other skin diseases that were once extremely common in people with HIV now occur far less frequently, thanks to new, more powerful antiviral drugs. If you have HIV and develop psoriasis (which can actually be one of the first signs of an HIV infection), there are many options for treating your condition.

Interestingly, antiviral drugs are the most commonly used therapy for psoriasis in people with HIV. The highly active antiretroviral treatment (HAART) for HIV usually controls psoriasis quite well in people who are HIV-positive, particularly if one of the HAART medications is an antiviral drug called azidothymidine (AZT). AZT often clears up psoriasis symptoms in people with HIV, but it doesn't appear to be as useful in people with psoriasis who are HIV-negative.

Because HIV-associated psoriasis can be quite severe, topical treatments aren't usually sufficient. Although vitamin D cream may be helpful if you have limited patches of psoriasis, UVB is the preferred choice in people with HIV and is considered not only effective, but also safe. Biologic treatments, except for alefacept, are another option if you have HIV, because they don't generally affect T-cell function significantly. Methotrexate is also a possibility, but drug interactions are more of a problem with this treatment.

There's no doubt that treatment choices are more complicated when you have HIV and drug interactions are a concern, so it may take some time, effort and research to find the treatment plan that's best for you. But you can take comfort in knowing that there are many more therapies and drug combinations available for people with HIV and psoriasis than ever before. Start by discussing your treatment options with your HIV physician and your dermatologist.

If You Have or Have Had Cancer

Because some psoriasis treatments can increase cancer risk or may cause existing cancers to grow more quickly, your doctor will probably use these treatments sparingly if you currently have or have had one or more malignancies. Although biologics (see page 85) are not the best option for you if you have a history of lymphoma, you can use them with caution even in this case if your doctor feels they are necessary.

If You're Having Surgery

You should let your dermatologist know if you're planning on having surgery. To reduce your risk of developing an infection, your doctor will probably ask you to stop taking any biologic medication you are on for a specific period before and after your operation. Although the studies that support this recommendation were done in people with rheumatoid arthritis, most physicians will choose to be safe and discontinue your psoriasis treatment temporarily.

If you need emergency surgery, don't worry about stopping your treatment ahead of time. However, it is important to let your surgeon and everyone else involved with your care know which psoriasis medications you're taking as soon as you can.

Discontinuing Biologics Before Surgery [MORE DETAIL]

The number of days you need to be off your biologic medication before surgery is determined by how long it takes for each drug to leave your system. As a rough estimate, your doctor may suggest discontinuing a biologic for at least three to five times the drug's half-life in your body. For the anti-TNF drugs, this means:
- Etanercept: 12 days (half-life 72 to 132 hours)
- Infliximab: 39 days (half-life 240 hours, or 10 days)
- Adalimumab: 56 days (half-life 10 to 20 days)

Getting Vaccinations

Vaccinations have the potential to be less effective and less safe if they're combined with systemic psoriasis treatments, because all of these drugs modify your immune system. It depends which drug you're on and whether the vaccine is "live" (meaning the virus or bacteria in the shot is alive), as opposed to being made from killed viruses or bacteria, or from completely non-infectious materials. The killed influenza and pneumococcus vaccines are safe while you are on any psoriasis treatment, but you may not receive their full benefits. Only about 10 percent of people get the full benefit of a killed vaccine if they are on cyclosporine, for example. (This is in contrast to people not on cyclosporine, where about 80 percent of people end up being protected.) If you're on a biologic drug, you'll have a 75 percent chance of being protected. If you're taking methotrexate, your odds of being protected are somewhere between 10 and 75 percent.

You should not get live vaccines, such as yellow fever, mumps, rubella and zoster (shingles), *at all* if you are on systemic psoriasis medications. The concern, in theory, is that because the psoriasis treatments block some of your immune functions, there is a risk that you will actually develop an infection from the live vaccine. Practically speaking, this is probably overcautious, because studies show that people on systemic medications continue to get the same sorts and severity of illnesses as other people.

As a precaution, you should discuss your situation with your primary care physician, your dermatologist and, if necessary, an infectious disease expert. As before surgery, you should stop taking your psoriasis medication three to five half-lives before receiving any vaccinations and restart your treatment about 4 weeks after being vaccinated to make the vaccination process as safe and effective as possible.

> **!** **[KEY POINT]**
>
> **Vaccines** that contain live viruses could theoretically trigger an infection in people on certain systemic psoriasis therapies. To be safe, your doctor will recommend that you receive only inactivated vaccines, and that you get all of your necessary shots before you begin biologic therapy.

Chapter 13

helping a child with psoriasis

What Happens in This Chapter
- Helping your family cope
- What psoriasis is like in children
- Treatment options for children
- How to make treatment time easier
- Handling bullies and when to seek professional counseling
- Other ways to improve your child's health

If your child is diagnosed with psoriasis, many treatment options are available, including topicals and systemic drugs. However, there's more to caring for your child than providing medication or visiting the doctor. It's important to educate your child about psoriasis and get support. Creating a plan to help your family adjust, involving your child in extracurricular activities, and teaching your child how to handle bullies and comments about his or her skin are also important. It's a good idea to make sure that your child's overall health is sound, as well.

Introduction

Caring for a child with a chronic (long-term) disease puts a huge strain on the whole family, emotionally and physically. In this chapter, we'll aim to take some of the worry and stress out of helping a child with psoriasis. We'll outline the main therapies for children with this condition, give you tips on how to make treatment time easier for you and your child, and provide you with guidance on how to help your child through some of the emotional struggles he or she might face.

Remember that the severity, extent and duration of your child's psoriasis are impossible to predict, so it's important to remain flexible, calm and positive. Although you will be anxious and want the best for your child, a great attitude will help you build a strong relationship with your child's healthcare team—if anything unexpected happens, you'll need them on your side. Most importantly, don't lose hope. More therapies are available for children than ever before, and more are being developed.

Your Child Has Psoriasis—Now What?

It can feel overwhelming to hear that your child has psoriasis. Although many parents are relieved to have a firm diagnosis at last, you might initially feel a bit lost or sad. You might also feel angry, guilty or shocked. It's okay to take some time to process these feelings and deal with them (see Chapter 11). Then, once you get your feet under you, there are a few things you can do to prepare for your child's psoriasis journey.

Educate Yourself, Your Child and Others in Your Child's Life

As soon as your child is diagnosed with psoriasis, we recommend that you learn about this condition, but take it slowly—too much information at once can be overwhelming. Start with Chapter 1 of this book, and then feel free to ask your doctor questions, talk to other parents who are coping and read additional books and articles about psoriasis in children.

Education is one of your best allies in helping your family and your child navigate the weeks, months and years ahead. Reading this chapter will give you most of the basics. You might also want to review the Resources section in the back of this book for more ideas on where to turn for information and support.

Once you understand more about psoriasis, you can tell your child about it. Use simple, straightforward language, and don't get too technical if your child is very young. Try a short explanation like, "You have something called psoriasis. You were born with it so it's not your fault that you have it. It means that your skin might sometimes get red, flaky and uncomfortable, but no one else can catch it. You can still go to school and have fun with your friends." Ensuring that your child is informed about psoriasis will help ease his or her fears and make it easier to handle challenging situations, such as treatments, teasing and making new friends.

> **! [KEY POINT]**
>
> **It's important** to let your child know that psoriasis doesn't define who he or she is—it's just a condition that he or she happens to have. Of course, this is much easier said than done. There is no question that psoriasis limits opportunities and has a large social, psychological and physical impact. Keep reading this chapter for tips on how to help your child build confidence and self-esteem.

You should also learn as much as you can about which triggers cause your child to flare (see Chapter 14) so that you can try to avoid them and come up with a plan for dealing with them. This will become more clear over time, as your child's disease progresses. For example, you might find that he or she gets worse with stress or after eating certain foods. Use the symptom diary at the back of this book (see page 228) to track changes in your child's symptoms and help you understand more about his or her flare patterns.

In addition, it's a good idea to educate others in your child's life, such as teachers, classmates, friends and extended family members. Making sure that the people who surround your child are informed about psoriasis will help reduce the chances of your child being teased or discriminated against. Educating those who are closest to your child to understand what it's like to have this condition is a key step in ensuring that he or she feels loved and supported.

Get Support

It's absolutely critical that your child has emotional support and that you don't underestimate the psychological impact of psoriasis.

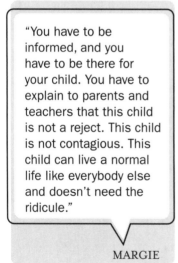

"You have to be informed, and you have to be there for your child. You have to explain to parents and teachers that this child is not a reject. This child is not contagious. This child can live a normal life like everybody else and doesn't need the ridicule."

MARGIE

People with psoriasis, including children, can feel suicidal if the pressures of their disease become too great, so making sure that your child has someone to talk to about his or her feelings can go a long way toward avoiding a crisis.

You don't necessarily need to send your child to a professional counselor (see How to Know When Your Child Needs Professional Counseling on page 197)—your child just needs to have someone to speak to, a person he or she trusts and feels comfortable with. This might be you, but don't be worried or hurt if it's someone else. It's normal for children to want to share their fears and challenges with people other than their parents. Your child might prefer to speak with an aunt or uncle, a grandmother or grandfather, someone at your family's place of worship, a best friend, a teacher, your family doctor or a pediatrician.

> "I think I had the best parents because they just stood by me and wouldn't let anybody say anything—and if they did they got put in their place. You have to protect [your kids]."
>
> MARGIE

Keep Communicating

If your child seems upset, don't let it slide. Ask what's wrong, and reassure your child that you are there to listen and be supportive. Try an opening line like, "You seem upset. What happened?" and be sure to tell your child that you love him or her and you want to help. Once you know what's wrong, you can decide whether or not you should seek professional counseling. If you're not sure what to do after talking to your child, it never hurts to ask your doctor for advice.

Get Your Child Involved in Activities

Participating in extracurricular activities can be an excellent way to build self-esteem. We recommend enrolling your child in a structured pastime that he or she enjoys, such as a choir group, a sports team or club, a scout pack, or a class such as dance, drama, ice-skating, cooking or art. Volunteering is also a good option. Your child will not only gain confidence and new skills by having a hobby, but will also develop a passion for life and strong friendships that will carry him or her through tough times.

Find a New Family Rhythm

When there is an illness in the family, it's easy for your world to get turned upside down. Your child's psoriasis could suddenly seem to be taking up most of your time and attention, and things like chores, caring for your other children, and your relationship with your spouse might take a back seat. It might take a while before you adjust to a new routine and find a new life balance, but try to talk with the members of your household about the challenges you're all facing. Come up with a plan for making your lives a bit easier. Maybe you can afford to eat out once a week instead of cooking? Maybe other family members can occasionally run errands for you? Work together as you adjust to your child's condition—and don't be afraid to ask for help.

> **!** **[KEY POINT]**
>
> **Encourage** brothers and sisters to be supportive of your sick child. It's an excellent way for them to learn how to be more sensitive to others and develop caregiving skills.

Be aware that your child may also start to ask for special treatment, such as skipping homework and chores or wanting to stay home from school when he or she isn't really sick. It will take some time and experience before you'll be able to tell when your child really is unwell and when he or she is just in need of some sympathy, reassurance and a little push to keep going with the daily routine. Don't let your child get away with dropping out of life or not following the rules just because he or she has a medical condition.

Teach Your Child How to Handle Comments

The psychological impact of psoriasis is often greatest in children because they are more vulnerable and just forming an image of themselves. That's why one the most important skills you can teach your child is how to handle comments made about his or her skin. Start by reviewing the kinds of questions people might ask (e.g., What's wrong with your skin? Is that contagious? Can I touch you? How did you get it? Are you all right?). Advise your child to answer in a relaxed and factual way, and then direct the conversation back to the situation at hand (e.g., I have a disease called psoriasis, but you can't catch it from me. I was born with it. Want to play on the swings with me?).

Practice to make sure your child is comfortable in all different kinds of scenarios, and emphasize that there's no need to become defensive or upset when a question comes up. Explain that people usually ask questions because they're curious, concerned, scared or surprised. Tell your child that if he or she stays calm and acts like psoriasis is no big deal, other people will also be at ease. For information on teasing, see Handling Bullies: How to Win the Unfair Fight on page 196.

What Is Psoriasis Like in Children?

There aren't a lot of firm statistics on the number of children with psoriasis, but estimates tell us that about one-third of people with this disease develop it before age 20. Psoriasis can actually appear in babies until age 2 in the form of psoriatic diaper rash, which looks like bright red plaques with clear borders. It often shows up in the groin and between the buttocks, as well as on the penis and labia. Other areas that children tend to develop lesions are the ears, elbows, knees, nails and scalp.

Be aware that scalp psoriasis can be mistaken for dandruff in children. Conversely, conditions that can look like psoriasis in young people include pityriasis rosea (a skin rash), eczema (see page 40) and candidiasis (see page 42).

There are some key differences between psoriasis in adults and children:

> "I got little heat spots around where my panties were on my waist. Some psoriasis [plaques] when you get them are really itchy and hot, and swell, so my mother thought maybe it's just the measles."
>
> MARGIE

- Psoriasis looks different in children—lesions are often thinner, smaller and less scaly, making this condition harder to diagnose in young people.
- Facial psoriasis and flexural psoriasis are more common in children.
- Psoriatic arthritis, which usually sets in some years after you first have psoriasis symptoms, is often not a problem in childhood.
- Psoriasis in children is triggered more often by external factors, such as injuries, drugs, physical trauma, stress or infections (e.g., tonsillitis, a cold or strep throat).

Making Psoriasis Manageable [MORE DETAIL]

Here are some ideas for making your child more comfortable when his or her psoriasis is flaring:

- Probably the most important thing you can do is work with your physician to find the best and most appropriate treatment (see Treatment Options for Children With Psoriasis on page 189)
- Help your child apply moisturizer frequently to reduce scaling and itching.
- Avoid hot baths and showers—they can increase itching.
- Keep your child's fingernails short.
- If the itching is too severe and short fingernails aren't doing the trick, it's sometimes better to let your child get a good sleep with a low dose of Benadryl (diphenhydramine) (be sure to ask your pediatrician, dermatologist or doctor before giving any medication to your child).
- Physical and emotional support will go a long way toward helping your child understand his or her disease, as will helping your child develop coping strategies (see Your Child Has Psoriasis—Now What? on page 182).

Treatment Options for Children With Psoriasis

Topical treatments (see Chapter 7) and conscientious skin care are often enough to allow your child to function normally and enjoy all the pleasures of growing up. Children are actually often more resilient than adults when it comes to tolerating treatments, but it's still important to monitor them carefully and engage them as much as possible in their treatment choices.

You should also make sure that your child is seeing a doctor who is very familiar with psoriasis medications used in children and their potential side effects. Your doctor will be able to guide you on which therapies are the best option for your child, so feel free to ask your physician lots of questions (see below).

Keep in mind that very few medications for treating psoriasis in children have been officially approved in children (only in adults) and, thus, are often used "off label." It is perfectly fine for your physician to use a drug off label; this is allowed if he or she thinks it will help your child. All it means in practice is that we don't know as much about the best dose and likely side effects in children, and your physician must use his or her clinical experience and knowledge to prescribe it safely.

Questions for Your Child's Doctor

Here is a list of questions that you might want to ask your child's doctor:
- What kind of psoriasis does my child have?
- Will this type of psoriasis go away?
- How common is this type of psoriasis, and how easy or hard is it to get under control?
- What are my child's treatment options?
- What kinds of side effects do these treatments have? What are their risks and benefits?
- How might this condition change with puberty or over my child's lifetime?
- What can trigger a flare?
- What types of changes in my child's condition are considered an emergency? How should I handle an emergency?
- How should I handle a non-emergency injury to my child's skin (e.g., cuts and scrapes)?
- What other kinds of non-skin-related symptoms should I be looking out for? If they appear, should I contact you immediately or wait until our next appointment?
- What should my child's daily skin care routine include?

- Are there any activities that my child should avoid?
- Do you know of any support groups for children with psoriasis?

Topical Treatments

Topical steroid creams (see page 69) are the first kind of treatment that your doctor will likely prescribe for your child. Physicians usually start with the lowest strength steroid that relieves a child's symptoms. If they prescribe a stronger steroid, they may advise less frequent use or switching to a milder steroid once the lesions begin to fade.

Calcipotriol (vitamin D cream—see page 71) is another topical medication used on children because it is not only effective, but also relatively safe. As in adults, one of its rarer side effects is higher-than-normal blood calcium levels, so regular monitoring while using this cream is required. Calcipotriol is also irritating to the skin, so it can't be used on a delicate area, such as the face.

Systemic Treatments

If your child's psoriasis isn't getting better with topical medications, don't worry—many other treatment options are available for young people. Although there aren't a lot of data on the use of systemic therapies in children, these more powerful treatments are sometimes used for severe cases. Each has its own set of benefits and drawbacks, and side effects are managed through careful observation. However, keep in mind that if you or your child has trouble following a treatment's instruction, your child should not be on that particular medication.

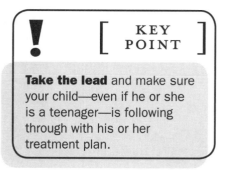

! **[KEY POINT]**

Take the lead and make sure your child—even if he or she is a teenager—is following through with his or her treatment plan.

Cyclosporine is usually well tolerated in children. However, because it can cause kidney damage and high blood pressure it is reserved for young people with the most severe cases of psoriasis, and it is generally used only for short periods of time. Methotrexate is also an option for children, although regular monitoring is required to check their liver function. The oral retinoid acitretin (see page 79) has been used successfully and safely in children, but long-term use of this medication can impair bone growth. Also, if your child is a girl in her teens, keep in mind that women need to be off acitretin for a full 3 years before it is safe for them to become pregnant.

Treatment	Benefits	Drawbacks
Cyclosporine	Well tolerated in children, with predictable side effects	Can cause kidney damage and high blood pressure
Methotrexate	Effective in children	Can cause liver damage, and reduced blood cell counts; reduces immune response to vaccines and infections
Acitretin	Effective in children	Can impair bone growth and harm a fetus; not very well tolerated at effective doses
Etanercept	The most-studied biologic in children and very effective, with predictable side effects (so we know what to expect)	Isolated cases of severe infections in adults only (i.e., not in children) and may be associated with a rare lymphoma when used with other, more powerful immunosuppressant drugs
UVB therapy	Effective and commonly used in children with psoriasis	Will increase risk of developing skin cancer with long-term use and should be used with caution in younger children

Of all the biologic drugs (see page 85), etanercept has been the most studied in children and can be very effective for treating 4- to 17-year-olds. A study published in 2008 found that children on etanercept started experiencing symptom relief within 4 weeks, and one-quarter of them experienced a 90 percent improvement in their PASI scores by week 12 of their treatment. In the end, half of the young people in this study saw a 75 percent improvement in their condition. This improvement was maintained for at least 36 weeks of treatment—in fact, these children responded better to etanercept than adults had in previous studies. Although some children had isolated cases of severe infection, etanercept appears to have the same basic set of side effects in children as it does in adults (see page 111).

Phototherapy is another option for young people with severe, extensive or treatment-resistant psoriasis, but it should be used with caution in younger children. Doctors usually try to limit a child's dose of UV rays because of the potential for cancer.

Making Treatment Time Easier

While some kids are pretty calm when facing the prospect of a needle, a doctor's visit or taking medicine, others can make quite a fuss. This happens because, unlike adults, children aren't used to compromising and aren't as capable of understanding that temporary pain or discomfort can help them feel better in the long run. Kids don't have your degree of life experience, and it can be hard for them to accept that a messy or uncomfortable treatment is actually for the best.

However, as stressful as it might be to see your child upset, know that resistance to treatment is very normal and there are ways to help make the experience easier (see Self-Help box on page 195). With enough love and persistence on your part, your child will eventually get used to treatments, and as he or she matures, you can start to encourage self-care so your child will be able to enjoy being independent as a teen and young adult.

Your dermatologist may also have some suggestions for helping your child use the medicine. Most dermatologists are very familiar with both the benefits and difficulties associated with applying creams, lotions, ointments and foams, and are usually able to help you make treatment time less stressful. Involving your child in the decision process regarding treatments can be another way to ensure that your child takes his or her medication.

Help Yourself— and Your Child— to Less Treatment Fuss

[SELF-HELP]

It might sound simple to follow your doctor's instructions to "simply apply the cream" to your child's psoriasis, but it's not uncommon for children to flat out refuse one or more of their prescribed therapies. Here are a few ways to make your child's treatments easier:

- Be sympathetic and acknowledge that the treatment isn't pleasant. Remember, even treatments that don't seem all that bad to adults can be scary to little kids.

- Educate your child so that he or she knows what to expect during and after the treatment (e.g., the cream might feel cold or sting, but then it will feel all right; it might feel uncomfortable and squishy, but it will make your skin feel better; the needle will pinch, but it doesn't hurt for very long).

- Consider giving a reward that is moderate and appropriate. For more uncomfortable and less frequent procedures, such as a needle, small children need immediate and tangible rewards, such as a new sticker for their collection or watching their favorite video. Older kids might get excited by a trip to their favorite restaurant, a visit to the zoo or a $5 donation toward something special they've been saving for. If your child receives daily treatments, you might want to give a reward at the end of each week or so, keeping track with a sticker chart.

- Provide lots of love and encouragement, but don't "over fuss" and pass your anxieties on to your child. If you're relaxed, patient and kind, you and your child will have a much easier time with the road ahead.

- Make sure life is as normal as possible while your child is undergoing psoriasis treatment.

Handling Bullies:
How to Win the Unfair Fight

Teasing is an unfortunate reality of life, especially if the target child is "different." Kids can be very mean, because they often aren't capable of accepting people who stand out in some way. Your child might have to face bullying, so it's important to teach him or her how to handle it and come through on top.

The best way to discourage bullies is to ignore them. However, this is much easier said than done. It's hard for children—or anyone—to ignore people who are saying mean or untrue things about them. The best way to try to prevent teasing from happening in the first place is to educate the kids in your child's class, as well as parents and teachers. If your child does report being teased, get the school and parents of the bullies involved right away—don't wait until the situation escalates. No amount of teasing is okay.

> "The kids at school, they didn't want to play with me because they thought it was contagious—they called me a leper."
>
> MARGIE

How to Know When Your Child Needs Professional Counseling

Your child might occasionally have a hard time with his or her psoriasis, and this is normal. But many parents wonder when to seek additional support. Even if your child isn't telling you outright that there's a serious problem, the clues listed below can be good indicators of when it's time to consult a professional counselor:

- Your child's overall mood has changed (e.g., he or she seems continuously anxious, angry, withdrawn, depressed or afraid).
- Your child's grades have slipped.
- Your child's behaviour has changed (e.g., he or she acts out or becomes defiant).
- Your child refuses to go to school or skips classes.
- Your child's sleeping patterns have changed.
- Your child's appetite has changed.

Don't be afraid to ask for help if you feel you can no longer handle the situation—there's no shame in seeking help when you need it!

Other Things to Do for Your Child's Health

Aside from love, support, community and some form of physical activity, feeding your child nutritious food is essential. Keep in mind that there's no such thing as "kid food"—children don't need pop, chips, pizza and hot dogs to enjoy eating. Read Chapter 10 for some healthy eating guidelines that will benefit your whole family, and you can find nutritious, simple recipes at www.yourpsoriasis.org

Chapter 14

all about flares

What Happens in This Chapter
- What a flare is
- What causes flares
- Avoiding flare triggers
- Treating flares

It can be frustrating if your psoriasis suddenly gets worse, or flares. But rest assured that there are ways to treat flares, as well as avoid what triggers them in the first place.

Introduction

If you've had psoriasis for a while, you've probably had a flare. Just when you feel your condition is under control, your symptoms start to return. You find yourself right back where you started, or even worse off. Although this frustrating experience is common in a recurring disease such as psoriasis, there are ways to manage and prevent flares, some of which have specific triggers that can be avoided.

Understanding Flares: Definition and Causes

A flare is what happens when your psoriasis gets worse or changes in nature. For example, you would be having a flare if the plaque psoriasis on your elbows suddenly spread to your trunk or you developed a new kind of psoriasis, such as pustular psoriasis. You can flare while you're on medication or off medication, or sometimes as a result of stopping a medication, which is also called a rebound. Flares are also sometimes called **exacerbations** (pronounced egg-za-sur-BAY-shonz).

> **[KEY POINT]**
>
> **It's very common** for psoriasis to change in severity over time, with most of these changes being minimal. However, more severe changes need to be addressed. Contact your doctor immediately if you notice that your symptoms are becoming much worse or changing. There are many ways to treat flares of all kinds.

Common Flare Triggers

What might make one person flare and not another is likely a combination of genetics, environment, health status and health history. Although some flare triggers are avoidable, many are not, and most vary from person to person. It will take some time for you to become familiar with your body's rhythms and figure out which triggers cause you to flare. Some of the most common triggers include:

- Physical trauma to the skin, such as an injury (e.g., cut, scrape or burn)
- Weather—due to less sun or UV exposure and dry air
- Strep infections
- Emotional stress—some people feel that emotional upheavals may trigger their flares
- Delivering a baby—a lot of women find that being pregnant causes their psoriasis to either get worse or better, and giving birth may lead to a return of psoriasis after many months of good control
- Sudden withdrawal of your psoriasis medication—in some people, stopping corticosteroids, creams or tablets, will cause a rebound (e.g., people who stop taking cyclosporine can develop generalized pustular or erythrodermic psoriasis)
- Certain drugs, such as lithium, which is the only medication consistently associated with a worsening of psoriasis; however, lithium is a very useful medication and it may not be necessary for you to stop taking it because you get psoriasis—just be sure to get your psoriasis treated while you're on this drug

Smoking and drinking alcohol are two other possible flare triggers. A lot of people with severe psoriasis are heavy smokers and drinkers. Although you could argue that it is the extreme physical discomfort and depression that are driving them to smoke and drink, I (Kim Papp) have noticed in my practice that the psoriasis of heavy drinkers is harder to treat. When they reduce or stop their alcohol consumption, their psoriasis is much more responsive to therapy.

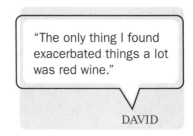

"The only thing I found exacerbated things a lot was red wine."

DAVID

Interestingly, a Finnish study published in 1990 in the *British Medical Journal* seems to back up this observation. Researchers found that men with psoriasis not only drank more alcohol than men with other skin conditions, but these men also reported that drinking made their psoriasis worse. Doctors at the Harvard Medical School and the Harvard School of Public Health found that women who drink non-light beer are more likely to develop psoriasis.

Smoking may also directly affect your skin. A group of scientists in Korea discovered that cigarette smoke increases the output of chemicals that cause skin inflammation. A small study conducted on people with palmoplantar psoriasis published in the *Journal of the American Academy of Dermatology* in 2006 showed that when participants stopped smoking, their condition improved significantly. A study published in 2004 in the *International Journal of Dermatology* found that people with psoriasis who smoked cigarettes had higher Psoriasis Disability Index and Psoriasis Life Stress Inventory scores.

Regardless of the evidence linking psoriasis severity to drinking and smoking, it's best to stop these harmful habits to stay as healthy as you can. Of course, that's much easier said than done, but it is possible to make major lifestyle changes, even if you have to try more than once. Be patient and kind with yourself. It can take a while to undo habits that have developed over a lifetime.

You don't have to face your journey to quitting alone—there's lots of support. For information on quitting smoking and drinking, see the Resources section at the back of this book. For information on appropriate ways to deal with chronic pain and depression, talk to your doctor and see page 163.

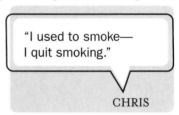

"I used to smoke—I quit smoking."

CHRIS

Avoiding Flare Triggers: You're More in Control Than You Think

When you flare, it's normal to feel a bit helpless. However, as you get to know your own body and which triggers cause you to flare, you can start learning how to avoid making your psoriasis worse. For example, you can keep your stress in check (see Chapter 11), protect your skin from the cold and possible injury (see Self-Help box on page 203), and take good care of yourself to reduce your chances of catching an infection (see Chapters 8, 10 and 11).

As we discussed, reducing how much alcohol you drink and quitting smoking may also make a difference. In addition, your doctor will help you avoid flares by prescribing drugs to smooth your transition to new medications or off your current medication. However, if you think that one of your medications is making your psoriasis worse or you want to stop taking one of the drugs to treat your psoriasis, never stop without talking to your doctor first. Going off a drug suddenly can have dangerous side effects.

Use the symptom diary at the back of this book (see page 228) to track changes in your symptoms and what might be causing you to flare. Knowing more about the factors that are influencing the course of your disease will not only help you feel more prepared for the road ahead, but also improve the chances that your condition will stay under control.

Help Yourself to Fewer Flares

[SELF-HELP]

Here are a few simple ways to reduce your chances of triggering a flare by injuring or irritating your skin:

- Keep your fingernails short to prevent them from getting caught and injuring the skin underneath them.

- Because wet skin is easily irritated, keep your genitals and skin folds as dry as possible by using talcum powder, drying well after you bathe or shower, and wearing cotton underwear and loose-fitting slacks.

- Don't use cornstarch to absorb moisture on your skin because it can encourage yeast growth and lead to an infection.

Treating Flares: Relief Is Possible

There are many effective ways to treat exacerbations. If a drug is making your symptoms worse, you may be asked to stop taking it, or your doctor may replace it with another medication. Although there is very little you can do to avoid the hormonal changes that occur with the end of pregnancy, there are effective ways to treat exacerbations before, during and after pregnancy (see pages 171 to 174). And if the worst happens and you experience a very serious flare, many treatment options are available to get you through it.

> "[After] the [drug] got out of my system ... they call it 'blossoming.' [My psoriasis] blossomed for three-and-a-half weeks."
>
> MARGIE

Chapter 15

future directions in psoriasis treatment

What Happens in This Chapter
- Ever-rising expectations for better treatments
- New therapies on the horizon
- The far future—genetics, individualized therapy and vaccinations

Psoriasis treatment has come a long way since its early days. A wide range of greatly improved therapeutic options are now available, and more are on the way. Scientists are also investigating the genetics of psoriasis in the hope of offering individualized treatment plans one day.

We've Come a Long Way

There have been many developments in the understanding and treatment of psoriasis since the days when it was confused with leprosy. Researchers all over the world are finding new clues to the causes of this condition and new drug options to help control it. Also, more and more doctors are approaching the treatment of psoriasis in a way that is centered on the wishes and goals of people with this disease. From improved standards to exciting research directions, the future of psoriasis care is looking bright.

Standards of Care

One of the main developments in treating psoriasis is the principle that people with this condition have the right to more effective therapies and better control of their disease. The definition of successful treatment will soon no longer be determined by lab results and test scores alone—the subjective effects of the disease are becoming increasingly important. People with psoriasis are clearly starting to have more of a voice in their care, and physicians are being trained to listen to their patients' needs.

The meaning of effective therapy is also changing. In most psoriasis research, 75 percent improvement is considered a good response to treatment. In practice, most people with psoriasis used to be happy if they saw a 50 percent improvement in their condition, because the available therapies really couldn't deliver anything better. The newest therapies being researched will likely raise expectations to 90 percent or 100 percent improvement. Clinical trials are also being designed to look at the way psoriasis affects people's lives.

Whenever clinicians are trying to make decisions about how to meet the ever-increasing standards in the world of psoriasis treatment, they can now turn to the *Canadian Psoriasis Guidelines*, which are probably the best in the world. These *Guidelines* are available to everyone and help doctors select the best therapies for all kinds of people with psoriasis, including children, people with HIV and pregnant women.

New Therapies and Approaches

New medications are always being developed that may be safe and helpful for treating psoriasis. Voclosporin (related to cyclosporine) may be available in Canada soon. While voclosporin may interact with many medications, it could be more convenient to use than cyclosporine because the best dose to achieve control of your psoriasis may be easier to find. Two new oral medications, apremilast and tasocitinib, are still being tested as we write this book, but they may be available to doctors in the near future. Both are tablets designed to be taken once or twice a day, and both look promising, based on the evidence we've seen so far. Other interesting oral psoriasis drugs are the fumaric acid esters (FAEs), which have been used in Germany for many years. New research on FAEs will be conducted in Canada in the coming years because the original studies done on these drugs are not up to current standards.

New injectable biologic drugs—golimumab and briakinumab—may provide new options for patients. Golimumab is already available for treating psoriatic arthritis, and it can be very effective at controlling psoriasis skin symptoms, along with stiffness and pain in the joints. Golimumab is related to the other anti-TNF biologics and probably shares many of the same safety issues. Briakinumab is not yet in use, but it is similar to ustekinumab. As well, several new and very exciting potential therapies are now in research.

Meanwhile, there are still many hurdles to overcome, especially when someone is struggling with more than just skin symptoms. Some therapies are better at treating joints than skin, and vice versa. Furthermore, because no treatment works for everyone and, over time, most treatments stop working, it may still take several attempts and different therapies to find the one that's best for each person.

A Word from Dr. Papp

A Word About the Evolution of Psoriasis Treatments

I have been in practice for over 20 years and involved in research for over 18. When I first started out, treating psoriasis was very different to how it is now. Most of my patients seemed to do well with the creams available at the time, and a few would do well with phototherapy or methotrexate.

But I noticed that a lot of these people weren't coming back for their follow-up visits after 1 or 2 years. I would then see them years later and they would tell me that their therapies weren't working anymore, that their psoriasis was worse or that the treatments were never really effective. It was obvious that a lot of people with psoriasis weren't doing well on existing treatments.

When research on biologic drugs for psoriasis started, it was amazing. Many of my patients who'd had no luck with the other therapies finally got relief—they were so much better and so much happier than they had ever been. These new breakthroughs have given us a revolution in treating psoriasis. This is the main reason I continue to do research.

Every time we research a new therapy, we make new discoveries about psoriasis, how it affects people's lives and how to treat it better. We have come a long way, but I think we have much farther to go.

Future Research

Future psoriasis research is heading in some exciting directions.

More and more research is being done on how psoriasis treatments may provide additional benefits, beyond controlling skin disease. For example, people with psoriasis are more likely to have heart attacks or strokes or develop diabetes. We still don't know, but may soon learn, whether treating psoriasis early and effectively can prevent the development of these tag-along conditions.

Researchers are also beginning to explore how to use our improved understanding of the genetics of psoriasis to create individualized treatment plans. As we come to understand the genetics of psoriasis better, it may even become possible to prevent the disease in people who would be at risk of developing it, using some form of vaccination.

The medical community is constantly working on ways to make treatments safer and easier for people with psoriasis to use. There will no doubt be many advances in the near future that will make the lives of people struggling with this condition better. Stay hopeful, and keep talking to your doctor about new drug developments—you just never know when a big medical breakthrough will happen!

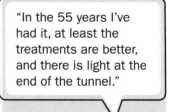

"In the 55 years I've had it, at least the treatments are better, and there is light at the end of the tunnel."

MARGIE

glossary

Acquired Immune Deficiency Syndrome (AIDS) a condition caused by the HIV virus, which leads to a failure of the immune system

Arthritis inflammation in the joints

Autoimmune disease a disease that causes the body to attack itself

Body Surface Area (BSA) measures the percentage of the body that is affected by psoriasis (measured in "palms" because the palm of the hand is about 1 percent of the total body surface area)

Blood pressure the force that blood exerts on the inner walls of the blood vessels as it flows through them

Biologics drugs that are produced by biological processes, such as genetic engineening

Candida a common yeast that can sometimes overgrow in or on the body; when it overgrows, it causes candidiasis

Cardiovascular disease (CVD) a term referring to diseases that affect the circulatory system (i.e., the heart, veins and arteries)

Celiac disease a condition in which the lining of the small intestine becomes damaged and cannot absorb nutrients properly. The damage is caused by the body reacting to gluten in food.

Cholesterol a substance that travels through the bloodstream and is important for producing hormones, synthesizing vitamin D, forming cell membranes and helping with fat digestion. Cholesterol travels in different kinds of packages: HDL is considered the "healthy" cholesterol. LDL is considered the "lousy" cholesterol because a high level of LDL is associated with greater risk of cardiovascular disease

Clinical trial a health-related study designed to test the safety and effectiveness of a treatment

Combination therapy a type of treatment that combines two or more therapies

Comorbidity a condition that can occur at the same time as another condition (e.g., depression is a comorbidity of psoriasis)

Crohn's diseae a digestive disease that can cause inflammation anywhere along the digestive tract

Dermatology Life Quality Index (DLQI) a questionnaire that allows you to rank your level of itch, pain and feelings of embarrassment/self-consciousness, note any problems with treatment, and rate how much you feel your condition is interfering with daily activities, relationships and sex; scores range from 0 (no impairment) to 30 (worst impairment)

Diabetes a disease that affects the body's production of insulin, a hormone that regulates blood sugar; type 1 occurs when the immune system destroys the cells that make insulin, and type 2 occurs when the body can't make enough insulin

Eczema a skin condition that is sometimes mistaken for psoriasis

Erythrodermic psoriasis a type of psoriasis that affects the entire body and sometimes requires hospitalization

Exacerbation a worsening of symptoms

Flare a worsening of symptoms while on a treatment

Gluten a protein component of certain grains, such as rye, barley, wheat, spelt and kamut

Goal a desired achievement (e.g., controlling your psoriasis by your next birthday)

Guttate psoriasis a type of psoriasis that develops after a streptococcal infection; characterized by small, coin-sized patches on the trunk, arms, legs and face

Hepatitis a virus that attacks the liver cells (hepatocytes)

Hormone a chemical messenger in the body

Human immunodeficiency virus (HIV) a virus that weakens the immune system by attacking a type of white blood cell, causing acquired immune deficiency syndrome (AIDS)

Inflammatory bowel disease an umbrella term for two conditions: Crohn's disease and ulcerative colitis

Leprosy a contagious disease caused by bacteria and was once confused with psoriasis (interestingly, the least contagious infection known)

Lesion a red, raised, scaly patch of psoriasis

Lupus a chronic disease that causes inflammation in many parts of the body

Medicare the term for Canada's healthcare system

Meditation an ancient practice that calms and focuses the mind

Metabolic syndrome a term used to describe a group of symptoms that occur simultaneously: obesity, elevated insulin levels, high blood pressure and high cholesterol

Mild psoriasis psoriasis that is treatable with topical medication and has a minimal impact on your quality of life

Moderate psoriasis psoriasis that isn't controlled well through routine skin care and significantly affects quality of life

Obesity an excessive amount of body fat

Oral treatments treatments that are taken by mouth, such as pills

Papule an elevated lesion that is smaller than 0.5 cm in diameter

PASI Change a severity rating tool that tracks how much psoriasis has changed in severity

Phototherapy a type of treatment that involves exposing the body to UVA and UVB lights

Physician's Global Assessment (static PGA and dynamic PGA) the static PGA assesses how severe your disease is at one point in time; the dynamic PGA assesses your response to treatment

Plaque a lesion that is larger than 0.5 cm in diameter

Plaque psoriasis the most common type of psoriasis, characterized by red, scaly, itchy, raised lesions that are at least 0.5 cm in diameter

Progressive muscle relaxation a relaxation technique that requires you to tense and then release all of your muscles, one by one

Psoriasis a chronic, lifelong, recurring, inflammatory, non-contagious skin condition

Psoriasis Area and Severity Index (PASI) a severity rating tool that allows a doctor to score the thickness, redness and scaling of psoriasis, as well as how much of the body surface and which areas of the body are affected; scores range from 0 (no disease) to 72 (worst disease)

Psoriatic arthritis a type of arthritis that can occur along with psoriasis

Pustular psoriasis a type of psoriasis that is often triggered by stress, smoking, infections and certain medications; characterized by small, raised blisters filled with non-infections pus surrounded by red skin; can be localized on the hands and feet or generalized over the entire body

PUVA a type of psoriasis treatment that combines psoralin and UVA light therapy

Ringworm a type of fungal infection that can be mistaken for psoriasis

Short Form (SF-36) Health Survey a general quality-of-life rating tool that is not specific to psoriasis or dermatology; it asks about pain, as well as about general perceptions of health, vitality, social functioning and mental health

Seborrheic dermatitis often associated with dandruff; appears as red patches with waxy scale and is commonly found on the scalp, ears and central face

Severe psoriasis psoriasis that isn't controlled well through topical treatments and causes an extreme reduction in quality of life

Side effect an unintended change in the body caused by any external intervention, such as medicine

Sign an objective measure showing change in the body (e.g., redness of skin)

Skin biopsy a medical procedure that involves taking a sample of skin to examine under a microscope

Strategy an overarching plan that allows you to achieve your goals

Symptom a perceived change in health status (e.g., feelings of depression, more itching)

Systemic treatments treatments that are taken by mouth (pills), suppositories or injection

Teratogenic capable of harming a fetus, causing abnormal growth

Topical treatments treatments that are applied to the skin, such as creams, sprays, gels and lotions

Toronto Psoriatic Arthritis Screen (ToPAS) a patient self-assessment tool to help detect the presence of psoriatic arthritis

Ulcerative colitis a digestive disease that causes inflammation and ulceration in the colon

Vegan a style of eating that eliminates all animal products from the diet (e.g., honey, eggs, meat, fish, dairy)

Vegetarian a style of eating that eliminates meat and fish from the diet but retains honey, eggs and dairy products

Visualization a relaxation technique that requires you to imagine positive imagery

Yoga an ancient practice that involves holding specific physical postures to improve strength, balance and focus

resources

Find The Canadian Guide to Psoriasis *supplementary materials online at www.yourpsoriasis.org*

Canada's Healthcare System and Health Benefits

Canada Benefits
Tel: 1–800-622-6232
TTY/TDD: 1-800-926-9105
www.canadabenefits.gc.ca

Communities Achieving Responsive Services (CARS)
(for residents in rural or remote areas, or in Northern Canada)
Rural Voices, General Delivery
Longbow Lake, ON
P0X 1H0
Tel: 1-807-548-2114
Fax: 1-807-548-7730
ruralvoices@xplornet.com
www.carsprocess.com
http://ruralvoices.cimnet.ca

Health Canada
Address Locator 0900C2
Ottawa, ON
K1A 0K9
Tel: 613-957-2991
Toll-free: 1-866-225-0709
Fax: 613-941-5366
TTY: 1-800-267-1245
info@hc-sc.gc.ca
www.hc-sc.gc.ca/index-eng.php

Non-Insured Health Benefits for First Nations and Inuit
www.hc-sc.gc.ca/fniah-spnia/
nihb-ssna/index-eng.php

Provincial and Territorial Drug Benefits
www.hc-sc.gc.ca/hcs-sss/pharma/acces/ptprog-eng.php

Clinical Trials

International clinical trial information
www.clinicaltrials.gov

Probity Medical Research Inc.
Clinical trial information
139 Union Street East
Waterloo, ON
N2J 1C4
Tel: 519-576-0768, ext 0
studies@researchtrials.org
www.researchtrials.org
www.probitymedical.com

Disease Education and Emotional Support

Psoriasis and Arthritis Groups

Canadian Skin Patient Alliance
2446 Bank Street, Suite 383
Ottawa, ON
K1V 1A8
Tel: 613-224-4266
Fax: 613-422-4267
www.skinpatientalliance.ca

National Psoriasis Foundation
6600 SW 92nd Avenue, Suite 300
Portland, OR
97223-7195
U.S.A.
Tel: 503-244-7404
or 1-800-723-9166
Fax: 503-245-0626
getinfo@psoriasis.org
www.psoriasis.org

PsoriasisPatients.com
www.psoriasispatients.com

Psoriasis Society of Canada
P.O. Box 25015
Halifax, NS
B3M 4H4
Tel: 1-800-656-4494
Fax: 902-443-2073
www.psoriasissociety.org

The Arthritis Society
393 University Avenue
Suite 1700
Toronto, ON
M5G 1E6
Tel: 416-979-7228
Fax: 416-979-8366
info@on.arthritis.ca
www.arthritis.ca

Counselors, Psychotherapists, Psychologists and Therapists

Canadian Counselling and Psychotherapist Association
www.ccpa-accp.ca/en/findcounsellor

Canadian Professional Counsellors Association
www.cpca-rpc.ca/counsellor-directory

Psychology Today—
Find a Therapist
http://therapists.psychologytoday.com/rms

Registry of Marriage and Family Therapists in Canada Inc.
www.marriageandfamily.ca

Meditation, Inspiration and Stress Reduction

A Tidewater Morning by William Styron

Eventide by Kent Haruf

Full Catastrophe Living by Jon Kabat-Zinn

Goodbye to a River by John Graves

On Death and Dying by Elisabeth Kübler-Ross

Oyster by John Biguenet

Plainsong by Kent Haruf

Stress Management for Dummies by Allen Elkin

Why Zebras Don't Get Ulcers by Robert Sapolsky

Health and Beyond Guided Meditation CDs
www.carolinedupont.com

How to Meditate by Lawrence LeShan

Mindfulness Meditation Practice CDs and Tapes
www.mindfulnesstapes.com

Healthy Eating

Nutrition Professionals

Dietitians of Canada—
Find a Dietitian
www.dietitians.ca/Find-A-Dietician/
Search-FAD.aspx

Holistic Nutrition Forum
Find a Holistic Nutritionist
www.holisticnutritionforum.com/
categories/Find-a-Holistic-Nutritionist

Cookbooks

Gluten-Free Cooking for Dummies
by Danna Korn and Connie Sarros

*Grain-Free Gourmet: Delicious Recipes
for Healthy Living*
by Jodi Bager and Jenny Lass

Enlightened Eating
by Caroline Dupont
www.carolinedupont.com

*Everyday Grain-Free Gourmet: Breakfast,
Lunch and Dinner*
by Jodi Bager and Jenny Lass

Healthy Sin Foods by Joey Shulman

How to Cook Everything Vegetarian
by Mark Bittman

Meals that Heal Inflammation
by Julie Daniluk

Healthy Eating Resources

Food Rules: An Eater's Manual
by Michael Pollen

Canada's Food Guide
www.hc-sc.gc.ca/fn-an/food-guide-
aliment/index-eng.php

Canadian Celiac Association
5025 Orbitor Drive
Building 1, Suite 400
Mississauga, ON
L4W 4Y5
Tel: 905-507-6208
Toll-free: 1-800-363-7296
Fax: 905-507-4673
info@celiac.ca
www.celiac.ca

Canadian Vegetarian Association
www.canadianvegetarian.org

**Environmental Defense Fund
Seafood Selector**
www.edf.org/page.cfm?tagID=1521

Grain-Free Gourmet Online
www.grainfreegourmet.com

Exercise

Canada's Physical Activity Guide
www.phac-aspc.gc.ca/hp-ps/hl-mvs/
pag-gap/index-eng.php

**International Taoist Tai Chi Society
and Taoist Tai Chi Society of Canada**
134 D'Arcy Street
Toronto, ON
M5T 1K3
Tel: 416-656-2110
headoffice@taoist.org
www.taoist.org

Yoga Directory Canada
1857 Florida Ave
Ottawa, ON
K1H 6Y9
Tel: 613-523-0825
info@yogadirectorycanada.com
www.yogadirectorycanada.com

Ahimsa Yoga
440 Bloor Street West, 2nd floor
Toronto, ON
M5S 1X5
Tel: 416-922-YOGA (9642)
info@ahimsayogacentre.com
www.ahimsayogacentre.com

Quit Smoking and Drinking

Quit Smoking

Quit 4 Life
(for teens aged 14 to 19)
www.quit4life.com

On the Road to Quitting Program
www.hc-sc.gc.ca/hc-ps/tobac-tabac/
quit-cesser/now-maintenant/road-
voie/index-eng.php

Quit Smoking Aids
www.hc-sc.gc.ca/hc-ps/tobac-tabac/
body-corps/aid-eng.php

The Lung Association – How to Quit Smoking
www.lung.ca/protect-protegez/
tobacco-tabagisme/quitting-cesser/
how-comment_e.php

Smoker's Helpline (Ontario)
Tel: 1-877-513-5333

Canadian Cancer Society
(British Columbia)
Tel: 1-877-455-2233
TTY: 1-888-445-5788
www.quitnow.ca

Canadian Cancer Society
Cancer Information
(Alberta/Northwest Territories)
Tel: 1-888-939-3333

Quit Drinking

Al-Anon and Alateen
Capital Corporate Centre
9 Antares Drive, Suite 245
Ottawa, ON
K2E 7V5
Tel: 613-723-8484
Fax: 613-723-0151
wso@al-anon.org
www.al-anon.alateen.org

Volunteer

Volunteer Canada
353 rue Dalhousie Street,
3rd Floor
Ottawa, ON
K1N 7G1
Tel: 613-231-4371
Toll-free: 1-800-670-0401
Fax: 613-231-6725
volunteercentres@volunteer.ca
vwww.volunteer.ca

CanadianAlliance for Development Initiatives and Projects (CADIP)
353-1350 Burrard Street
Vancouver, BC
V6Z 0C2
Tel: 604-628-7400
Fax: 604-998-1356
www.cadip.org

For Kids and Parents Whose Kids Have Psoriasis

Parenting Children With Health Issues
by Foster W. Cline and Lisa C. Greene
www.parentingchildrenwithhealthissues.com

**National Psoriasis Foundation's Site
for Kids With Psoriasis**
www.PsoMe.org

Scouts Canada
Tel: 1-888-SCOUTS-NOW
helpcentre@scouts.ca
www.scouts.ca

KidSport Canada
180-3820 Cessna Drive
Richmond, BC
V7B 0A2
Tel: 604-333-3650
Fax: 604-333-3450
www.kidsportcanada.ca

**1-2-3 Magic: Easy-to-Learn
Parenting Solutions**
www.parentmagic.com

Parenting children with Health Issues
by Foster W. Cline and Lisa C. Greene
www.parentingchildrenwithhealthissues.com

your diary

MY PSORIASIS HISTORY

My age of psoriasis onset_____

_____

Where my psoriasis occurs_____

_____

_____

My symptoms (e.g., joint, skin)_____

_____

_____

_____

Find The Canadian Guide to Psoriasis *supplementary materials online at www.yourpsoriasis.org*

MY HEALTH AND PERSONAL HISTORY

Age_____

Occupation_____

Place of birth_____

Major surgeries_____

_____

_____

Major childhood illnesses_____

_____

Other major health events or illnesses

(e.g., accidents, heart attacks)_____

_____

_____

Vaccinations received _____

_____

_____

History of smoking and alcohol consumption_____

_____

Ongoing infections (e.g., hepatitis or HIV)_____

_____

_____

Previous tests for tuberculosis_____

BCG vaccine history_____

Exposure to tuberculosis_____

FAMILY PSORIASIS HISTORY

Others in my family who have or have had psoriasis_____

_____

Where their disease occurs_____

_____

Their symptoms (e.g., joint, skin)_____

_____

FAMILY HEALTH HISTORY

Family members who had a heart attack or stroke before
age 60 _____

_____

Number of parents and siblings with multiple sclerosis

_____

TEST AND RESULTS

Test	Date	Result

PSORIASIS TREATMENTS

Treatment	Date	Results

OTHER MEDICATIONS AND SUPPLEMENTS

Medication or supplement_____

Reason taking_____

Medication or supplement_____

Reason taking _____

Medication or supplement _____

Reason taking _____

APPOINTMENTS

Date_____

Time_____

Location _____

Date_____

Time_____

Location _____

Date_____

Time_____

Location _____

Date_____

Time_____

Location _____

Date_____

Time_____

Location _____

APPOINTMENTS

Date_____

Time_____

Location _____

_____

Date_____

Time_____

Location _____

_____

Date_____

Time_____

Location _____

_____

Date_____

Time_____

Location _____

_____

Date_____

Time_____

Location _____

_____

IMPORTANT CONTACTS

In an emergency call _____

Doctors _____

_____

_____

Therapists _____

_____

_____

Pharmacist/pharmacy _____

_____

JOURNAL

index